A Toddler's Tale:
Life In Lockdown

# A Toddler's Tale: Life In Lockdown

AARON J. BUCKLEY

Copyright © 2025 Aaron J. Buckley

The moral right of the author has been asserted.

Apart from any fair dealing for the purposes of research or private study, or criticism or review, as permitted under the Copyright, Designs and Patents Act 1988, this publication may only be reproduced, stored or transmitted, in any form or by any means, with the prior permission in writing of the publishers, or in the case of reprographic reproduction in accordance with the terms of licences issued by the Copyright Licensing Agency. Enquiries concerning reproduction outside those terms should be sent to the publishers.

Troubador Publishing Ltd
Unit E2 Airfield Business Park
Harrison Road, Market Harborough
Leicestershire LE16 7UL
Tel: 0116 279 2299
Email: books@troubador.co.uk
Web: www.troubador.co.uk

ISBN 978 1 83628 225 9

British Library Cataloguing in Publication Data.
A catalogue record for this book is available from the British Library.

The manufacturer's authorised representative in the EU for product safety is Authorised Rep Compliance Ltd, 71 Lower Baggot Street, Dublin D02 P593 Ireland (www.arccompliance.com).

Printed and bound in Great Britain by 4edge Limited
Typeset in 11pt Minion Pro by Troubador Publishing Ltd, Leicester, UK

## Dedication

Firstly I would like to thank the central character in this book, my eldest son Noah. Your personality and quirks inspired me to start writing a diary in March 2020. I never intended for the collection of seven diaries to be typed up, let alone published. My love for you meant that I could not put the pen down when, at times, it would have been easier to do so.

Thanks to my wife, Stacie, for all your love and support. Thanks for giving me the space and time to write this book. I know at times you would rather I had been doing something else to support our hectic family life, parenting three boys.

Thanks to my friends Jon and Kieran. Jon, for giving me the motivation to type the diaries up after you had read the first three thousand words. You were the first person outside of my family to give me the confidence and belief that this book was possible. Kieran, thanks for your help with my website. Information Communication Technology is not my strong point and your expertise alleviated my anxieties tremendously!

And thanks to you, for buying this book! I hope you enjoy.

Chapter 1

# BEFORE EVERYONE WAS TOLD TO 'STAY AT HOME'

**21st December 2019**
The first people in China were treated for 'pneumonia of an unknown cause'. This was not reported to the rest of the world until 20th January 2020.

**31st December 2019**
Doctors in China continue to treat lots of people for 'pneumonia of an unknown cause'. Early in the New Year, Chinese researchers identified a new virus that had infected lots of people. They did not know that this virus could be spread by humans.

**11th January 2020**
The first person in the world died of Covid-19 in Wuhan, China.

**20th January 2020**
The first cases of Covid-19 were reported outside of China. These were in Japan, South Korea and Thailand.

**29th January 2020**
The first two cases of Covid-19 were reported in the United Kingdom.

**30th January 2020**
The World Health Organisation (WHO) declared a global health emergency in respect of Covid-19.

**7th February 2020**
Li Wenliang, the Chinese doctor who was prevented from announcing the full, potential severity of the virus, died of Covid-19.

**11th February 2020**
Today, the virus was officially named 'Covid-19'. It stands for 'coronavirus disease'.

In China, 1,113 people have now died from the disease and there have been 44,653 cases of infection.

There have been 393 cases of Covid-19 outside of China.

**28th February 2020**
The first British person died of Covid-19, on board a cruise ship in Japan.

The Government confirmed the first case of Covid-19 to be passed on inside our country.

**2nd March 2020**

An Italian doctor tested positive for Covid-19 at the H10 Costa Adeje Palace in Tenerife, where people have to now isolate in their room. Your Grandma and Grandad Buckley stayed in the same hotel just over a week ago!

**10th March 2020**

Six people have now died from the virus in the UK, with 373 others testing positive.

**11th March 2020**

The WHO declared Covid-19 a pandemic. A 'pandemic' is the word used for a disease which has spread around the world.

**12th March 2020**

I watched Manchester United for what would be the last time in months. They won 5–0 in their Europa League Round of 16 first leg tie against LASK Linz in Austria. The game was played in an empty stadium, with no fans in attendance.

**13th March 2020**

The English Premier League suspended football until at least 4th April 2020.

**14th March 2020**

The worry about the Covid-19 virus reaches our family. Due to age and different health conditions, your three great-grandparents: Mave, Anne and Mike, and Grandad Ste and Aunt Stevie are all at heightened risk if they contract the virus.

**15th March 2020**
It was your friend Eric's little brother Arthur's christening at the cricket club. The atmosphere was strange and lots of people did not attend due to being worried about the virus. Oblivious to the changing world around us, you ate lots of cake and spent the afternoon kicking balloons around on the stage!

**16th March 2020**
Our Prime Minister Boris Johnson gave the first of what would end up being very regular briefings from Downing Street. The severity of the situation is becoming apparent as he asks everybody to work from home, avoid bars and restaurants and stay at least two metres away from others in public. The latter – 'social distancing' – is one of the terms that became part of our everyday language as we moved through the pandemic.

There is grave concern that the NHS is going to struggle to cope with the demand for treatment and care. Fifty-five people have now died and there have been 1,543 confirmed cases in the UK. It is thought that 10,000 people may have been unknowingly infected with Covid-19.

**17th March 2020**
The *2020 UEFA European Football Championship* was postponed until next year.

**18th March 2020**
Every Wednesday, you and your cousin Darcie are looked after by Grandma and Grandad Buckley. Today ended up being the last time in a while.

The Government announced that most schools will close from Friday until further notice. We are moving into extremely uncertain times.

### 20th March 2020
My birthday!

*Don't want it to be Daddy's birthday!* you claimed as you sang 'Happy Birthday' to Auntie Emma who celebrated hers over a month ago!

You spent the day with Nana Roz as Mummy went to work at her school for the last time until further notice.

I played at Hillside Golf Club and drank my last draught pint for a while in the clubhouse afterwards. Shortly after I left Southport, the Government ordered all pubs, restaurants, gyms and other social venues to close.

We celebrated my birthday at home with family members but some chose not to come for fear of catching the virus.

At this point, there is still a hopeful tinge of denial as we move forward into the unknown.

### 21st March 2020
Your swimming lessons were cancelled. I managed to squeeze a round of golf in as outdoor sports have yet to be banned.

More and more people are choosing to stay at home and not socialise with others.

### 22nd March 2020
It was Mother's Day so you bought Mummy some beauty products and a *pretty* plant.

Walking to Uncle Liam's and Auntie Emma's house for tea, people crossed the road in order to maintain 'social distancing'. There was an eerie, deserted atmosphere on the streets and a sense that something momentous was about to happen.

**23rd March 2020**
As Mummy and I worked from home you attended nursery as normal. You were one of only two children there.

At 8.30pm Boris Johnson, told the country, 'You must stay at home.' We can now only leave our houses to buy food, exercise for an hour once a day or to go to work if we absolutely cannot stay at home.

The hairs on the backs of our necks stood on end as Mummy and I watched the news, processing the orders that signalled normal life had ceased. We were now in lockdown.

Worldwide, Covid-19 figures stand at more than 270,000 cases and 11,000 deaths.

Life as we know it is over for now and this is the tale of how you lived as a toddler throughout the strangest and most difficult period of the last eighty years.

Chapter 2

# ISOLATION PERIOD ONE

**24th March 2020**
That's it! No work, no nursery, no contact with family and friends. Mummy and I have to stay at home, work and simultaneously care for and entertain you for at least three weeks.

It was a lovely sunny day so our exercise was a walk to see the horses at the end of the street. You particularly liked the one in the *red coat*!

Who can think of a better time to start potty-training a two-year-old than at the start of a national lockdown? We quickly gave up because by lunchtime you had emptied your bladder four times on the kitchen floor!

**25th March 2020**
Prince Charles tested positive for Covid-19.

We took a longer loop on our daily walk in the hope that you would tire out and fall asleep… so we could work!

You shouted, *Grandma!* at a random woman sat in her back garden! You will not be seeing Grandma today, Little Man!

**26th March 2020**
Today, the lockdown restrictions became law after the Coronavirus Act 2020 was fast-tracked through Parliament. This basically gives the Government the power to do what it feels is necessary to prevent the virus from spreading.

Fitness videos are all the rage across the country. Getting you to join in with ours is hard work. As is having to answer *what you doing?* three hundred times a day!

Your nursery education has not worn off just yet and at teatime you treated us to a lovely rendition of:

*Dinner's coming, dinner's coming,*
*Are you ready? Are you ready?*
*Fingers off the table, fingers off the table,*
*Hands on knees, hands on knees!*

At 8pm, we joined in with people up and down the country as several households on our street clapped and cheered on their doorsteps for the NHS workers who are battling daily to tackle the virus.

**27th March 2020**
Boris Johnson tested positive for Covid-19.

The weather continued to be glorious and we entertained ourselves by log rolling down the hills at the back of our house. We could not do it for longer than an hour, though!

**28th March 2020**
It is the weekend but that means nothing when you are isolating from everyone in lockdown.

*The Snail and the Whale* is definitely your favourite thing to watch on television.

Video calls have quickly become the best way for people to communicate with the outside world. Mummy sent a 'Happy Birthday' video to your friend Esme which took a while because you were insistent on singing 'Happy Birthday' to Auntie Emma, Grandma and everyone else whose birthday it is not!

**29th March 2020**
Potty-training resumed and you performed on your plastic tub whilst video-calling Grandma and Grandad. The regime is going relatively well. It is proving more successful when you are naked from the waist down, as you do forget to find your potty when you have your underpants on!

You are becoming quite the domesticated toddler – polishing the fish tank, washing up and helping to paint the wall in the kitchen.

Your family are missing you, as you spoke to Nana Roz, James and Auntie Stevie and Uncle Simon on two separate video calls.

**30th March 2020**
I had to go into work and, in my absence, Mummy sent me a picture of you grinning with your hair in a bobble.

I called you at lunchtime and your candid answer when I asked what you were doing was, *Playing with my willy!* You drew a rainbow with Mummy and put it up in the front room window as a 'Thank you' to the NHS.

Four stickers have been added to your potty-training chart to go with the one you earnt yesterday at bedtime.

The 2020 Summer Olympics in Tokyo have been postponed until next year. It is beginning to become apparent that life will not revert back to normal for some time yet.

**31$^{st}$ March 2020**
Holding video meetings with work colleagues is a challenge with your constant interruptions. It is also not ideal when you are spending the majority of your day with no nappy on!

Getting on my shoulders has worked well bringing you back home from a walk. Today, you refused to leave the house without getting on them first!

Your local geography knowledge is improving and you are starting to take the lead on our daily strolls.

**1$^{st}$ April 2020**
Today was mine and Mummy's fourth wedding anniversary. You gave Mummy some flowers whilst singing 'Happy Birthday!' to her.

We saw three deer on our walk and you called them 'Darcie Doo', 'Daddy', 'Mummy', 'Grandma' and 'Grandad', which just so happens to be five names! Your nursery education is evidently wearing off!

Having reneged on your afternoon nap, you were put to bed early so Mummy and I could enjoy a bottle of champagne.

There was a further sporting cancellation as the Wimbledon Tennis Championships, scheduled for June and July, was removed from the 2020 calendar.

Today, 563 people died from Covid-19, which represented the country's highest daily loss of life so far.

### 3rd April 2020

Your nude antics whilst learning how to toilet on your potty received a mention from the director in the daily Covid-19 bulletin at my work.

Grandma and Grandad Buckley dropped some soup off for us at home. They have not seen you for twelve days. They were not allowed to come in the house so you had to speak to them from the front door as they were stood at the end of the drive.

The queues to enter the supermarket are starting to snake around the side of the building and through the car park. People are wearing masks and covering their mouths with scarves and coats. Everyone has to stand at least two metres apart, in keeping with the social distancing policy, to try and prevent the virus from spreading.

People are discovering innovative ways of socialising due to having to remain at home. Tonight, Mummy and I had a quiz with friends over a Zoom video conference. I must admit, I did not know what Zoom was three weeks ago!

The day-on-day death toll is rising. 569 people died yesterday, followed by 684 today. The situation we are living through is certainly serious.

**4ᵗʰ April 2020**
Our second weekend in isolation. I dropped a painting off which you had done for Grandma and Grandad but was not allowed to go into their house. It felt strange having to talk to my own parents from the end of the path. I also called at Darcie's to give her a Grow Your Own Vegetable set. You have got one too so you are going to have a competition to see who can grow the best vegetables!

Each piddle on the potty is followed by, *High five! On the side! Up above! Down below! Too slow!*

After our daily dose of walking – a staple of the lockdown diet – we settled down in front of the television to watch *The Virtual Grand National*. This was a computer-generated horse race, with the world famous steeplechase being unable to take place at Aintree.

Great-Grandma Buckley's dog Kally was put to sleep today. She was fourteen years old and had lived with Auntie Michelle and Uncle Chris since Great-Grandma Buckley died more than four years ago.

708 people died from the virus today, including a five-year-old child. So devastatingly sad.

**5ᵗʰ April 2020**
Your insistence on striving for perfection, attempting to complete tasks an average adult would find almost impossible, is causing you to have monumental emotional outbursts. One example includes stacking a tower and trying to knock it over, by kicking a football, at the first attempt.

Washing the cars turned into a water fight between us. This was after you insisted that watering the bushes and cleaning the road were tasks far more important than actually cleaning the vehicles on the drive.

The Government is considering banning daily exercise because people are not adhering to social distancing. Such news supports Mummy's feelings that things are going to get worse before they start to get better.

Our ninety-three-year-old Queen Elizabeth II gave a television address, only the fourth time in her reign that she has done so outside of her annual Christmas Speech. She said, 'Better days will return; we will be with our friends again; we will be with our families again; we will meet again.' Let us hope so.

### 6th April 2020

Today, we should have been going on holiday to Tenerife for ten nights. On reflection, it seems ludicrous how we harboured hope of being able to travel abroad when lockdown started. If you were not already, you are becoming quite the little character! It certainly takes both me and Mummy to keep you in check!

On our walk you developed a curious fondness for smelling cars as well as flowers! You constantly remind me that, due to not wearing wellies, I am not allowed to splash in puddles or walk through *thick, oozy, mud*, in reference to the book *We're Going On A Bear Hunt*.

The number of daily deaths from Covid-19 dropped to its lowest level in a week but we still have no idea what could be ahead of us.

In golf, the Open Championship was cancelled and will now take place at Royal St George's next year.

## 7th April 2020

Boris Johnson spent last night in intensive care after his Covid-19 symptoms worsened.

I went into work today and you stayed at home with Mummy. She kept you busy with morning exercises and a scavenger hunt. You came home with a dandelion, two daisies, a *spiky weaf* (leaf) and an empty snail shell.

854 people died from Covid-19 today, the highest total yet. It feels as though the record total of daily deaths is being broken each day. Scientists predict that the peak of coronavirus infections and deaths will occur on 17th April.

## 8th April 2020

Each morning we are welcomed by you bringing five muslin cloths and a dozen or so teddies into our bedroom and plonking them on our bed!

Nana Roz and James have to go for Covid-19 tests tomorrow as James has been suffering from symptoms of the virus for three days.

The isolation of lockdown has started to affect your sanity. You spent the majority of the walk chasing your silhouette and referring to it as a *shan-dow*!

You kept missing the ball playing cricket with me. I asked where your coordination had gone. This led to you dropping the bat and looking around the garden, arms outstretched, asking, *Where's my 'd'nation'?!*

The novelty of speaking to people on video calls is wearing off. It is almost as if you are starting to sense things are not normal and you are frustrated by not being able to see family and friends face to face.

We received a letter through the post from Boris Johnson, reinforcing the 'Stay at Home' message.

938 people died from the virus today, taking the total number of deaths nationwide to 7,097.

## 9th April 2020

The emotional impact of the lockdown is starting to take its toll on me. For the last few days I have felt depressed and emotionally flat as a result of being cooped up at home. Whilst this is nowhere near as serious as suffering the potentially deadly effects of Covid-19, it is an example of how isolation is impacting people's mental health.

It is difficult for Mummy and I to continue to work full-time as well as look after and stimulate you. This is made more problematic given that your comprehension of the turmoil the country has been thrown into is almost minimal.

You have changed so much in the last three weeks and your cheeky nature and sense of fun helps to keep our spirits up, especially since we do not know when life will return to normal.

With the lighter nights it is becoming more difficult for you to settle at bedtime. We clapped the nation's care workers at the front door which did little to help you fall asleep.

*Mummy? Daddy? Why you clappin'?* you enquired from between the spindles of the bannister on the stairs.

## 10th April 2020

Today is Good Friday, which would usually mark the start of a busy Easter Bank Holiday weekend. You said that you wanted to go to Grandma and Grandad's house. It is virtually impossible to explain why you cannot in a way that you will understand.

We have seen you grow so much in confidence over the last few weeks. You are constantly the leader on our walks. *Come on! This way! Mummy, Daddy… let's go!*

Your friend Eric called round at the front door of our house with his mummy to drop an Easter card off for you. You were very excited to see him!

You end most video calls with family by performing a 'Wuhan kiss', which involves an elbow tap on the phone screen followed by blowing a kiss. Perhaps not the most sensitive gesture in the wider context, admittedly. Especially when 980 people died from Covid-19 today. This was more than Italy, one of the worst-affected countries in the world, have had in a single day up to now.

## 11th April 2020

The hottest day of the lockdown so far as the temperature reached 19°C.

You are developing some peculiar habits, like wanting to take your muslin cloth – *star blanket* – everywhere with you. This includes spreading it out on your chair when you sit down to eat like some loose, baggy seat covering.

We took a picnic out on our walk and you fed the horses some carrots out of your hand.

You entertained yourself on the lawn playing football and you can now just about tolerate being tackled without letting your emotions get the better of you!

Someone dressed as the Easter Bunny was doing the rounds on our estate and they gave you a chocolate egg! It was a heart-warming gesture of societal spirit, especially when society has all but been erased.

James was confirmed as having Covid-19. He spent four days in bed at the start of the week but he is now starting to feel a bit better.

**12th April 2020**
Easter Sunday.

When you woke up, you searched the house for eggs that the 'Easter Bunny' had hidden for you. This resulted in you eating way too much chocolate before breakfast.

Liam, Emma and Darcie dropped your Easter presents off and they stayed for a while in the garden at a 'social distance'. This was not acceptable for our next-door neighbour who popped his head over the fence and reminded us all that we should not be together. It was an understandable sign of the fear and anxiety that has swept the country.

On our walk you saw some lambs and brought home a *very hungry caterpillar*. You like to reference things you read about in your books in real life.

When asked, you told me that the favourite part of your day was *seeing Darcie Doo-Doo*.

Today, the UK passed 10,000 deaths from the virus.

**13th April 2020**
Most mornings, you sing, *No more monkeys jumping on the bed!* whilst jumping on our bed.

You and I baked some buns which we were going to share with Mrs Arain, our neighbour over the back fence, until you sneezed in the mixture!

Your answer to our question of 'Do you need a wee?'

as you sit on the couch watching *The Land Before Time* with no nappy on is usually *no thanks!*

You had your first-ever painful encounter with a stinging nettle when we were out and spent the remainder of the walk clutching a crumbling dock leaf in your hand.

Mrs Arain and her family passed an Easter egg and a toy car – a Porsche 911 – over the fence to go with your *Lam-bo-geeny*. You were ecstatic!

**14th April 2020**
You spent the morning helping Mummy to jet wash outside whilst I was at work.

Whilst you are not too fond of the steep walk up the hill, you now manage to walk most of it on your own. You are assertive, demanding Mummy and I stay *on the path!* You are inquisitive – *What's that?* – and take a real interest looking at all the animals and flowers. Today we saw some goats and you held Daddy's hand as you walked along the top of a *wobbedy* (wobbly) wall.

You decided against having a nap so spent the majority of late afternoon becoming disproportionately frustrated with your toys!

The UK surpassed 12,000 deaths from Covid-19 today. The toll sadly continues to rise.

**15th April 2020**
You and Mummy went for a walk on your own as I had lots of work to do. It was a very hot day but you still demanded to wear your wellies!

You now talk to Mrs Arain, Jimmy, Kaiser and Saif most days over the back fence.

You regressed a touch with your potty-training, urinating on the couch as well as in the cupboard whilst pretending to be a *little dinosaur.*

## 16th April 2020

Your hair is wild and your legs are covered in bruises. Lockdown life is certainly taking its toll on your physical appearance!

The wellies were finally ditched and you left the house appropriately dressed for the weather in a T-shirt, shorts and trainers.

We walked a mile up the steep hill and back and added cows to the list of animals we have seen so far in lockdown. You stopped to speak to strangers and told them how interesting your walks are! They took care not to get too close to you for fear of catching the virus.

The Government announced that the lockdown will continue for at least another three weeks. This will take us to the 7th May. They have to be sure that the peak of Covid-19 infections has passed and that the NHS are able to cope with the demand before life can return to anything like normal.

So… that is twenty-three days of lockdown completed and it is going to be another twenty-one days before we are any clearer about what life will look like in the near-future.

We have noticed such a change in your character over the last few weeks. Your speech has developed significantly, you constantly ask questions (*What's that? What's that noise?*), you are bossy (*Come on! Phone away!*

*Put it in your pocket! This way!*) and you are kind of getting the hang of where you should and should not urinate!

At times it has been tough, which has not been your fault, but Mummy and I both agree that without spending almost every waking minute with you lockdown would be a whole lot tougher… and much less entertaining!

Chapter 3

# ISOLATION PERIOD TWO

**17th April 2020**
The sun is shining, like it has done for a large part of lockdown, but it is freezing!

Your interest in flowers, and weeds, is growing and you like blowing the seeds off dandelions!

Your memory is excellent and you remember where different things have happened at the different stages on all the walks we have been on over the course of the last month.

Mrs Arain and her family have noticed how much your language has developed and enjoy having conversations with you over the fence.

**18th April 2020**
Feeding horses, jumping in streams, sheepdogs working, walking on walls, the *deep dark wood* (a reference to *The Gruffalo*), a *narrow, gloomy cave* (another reference to the

book *We're Going On A Bear Hunt*), a fallen tree, *Where's Spike?* and *big water* (references to your favourite television programme *The Land Before Time*), Daddy's shoulders.

All those were things you either saw, did or said on our three-mile walk. At two years and four months old you did very well to walk two thirds of it on your own.

You almost managed to do your first poo on the potty but, unfortunately, you parted with it on the kitchen floor. This evoked an amusing amount of fascination from you! At first, you were scared by what your bowels had produced!

You fell backwards off the end of our bed after jumping around when you should have been speaking to Stevie and Simon on a video call. Fortunately, or perhaps unfortunately, you did not hurt yourself enough to learn to stop!

**19th April 2020**

Today, the plan was to walk around the reservoir, which is a short drive from our house, but you fell asleep in the car en route! We have certainly not had to worry too much about the price of petrol since the end of March.

Back at home you had an unlucky afternoon, with multiple accidents befalling you. I 'kicked' a football at your nose, Mummy 'kicked' the same thing at your head, the wind blew your cup of orange cordial all over you and you got jammed between the pouffe and couch, head first!

Before bed you sent a video to Carol, one of Grandma's friends, singing 'Happy Birthday' and then proceeded to kick your orange juice all over the carpet!

16,060 people have now passed away in hospital from

Covid-19. Slightly more encouraging is that the death total today – 596 – is the smallest in the last two weeks. Are things beginning to settle down? We hope so.

**20th April 2020**
Nana Roz went back to work today after her Covid-19 test on 17th April came back negative.

It is the start of another working week for me and Mummy, as the last two weeks have been the school holidays. Keeping you occupied and feeling content is a challenge, as you want one of us to play with you most of the time.

Mummy and I have jobs which fall in the category of essential workers. This includes NHS staff, social care workers, and those people that work in childcare or education. Those who are vital in making sure that people are fed and watered and kept warm and safe are also classed as essential workers.

Employers of workers who are non-essential are able to apply for money to pay their staff who are on furlough. These people cannot go to work and must stay at home. Those who are furloughed can be paid up to eighty percent of their wage without working. This is to save businesses so that they are still here once we are through this mess.

You made chocolate an incentive for doing a wee on your potty, which led to you doing four in fifteen minutes. Nice try!

Before your bath you proudly told us, *Noah's got a big willy!* What a statement to round off four full weeks in isolation!

**21st April 2020**
The lack of driving we have done in the last four weeks has led to you growing a dislike for travelling in the car. I took you for a drive to drop some things off at a house for work and, *Don't want to do a job! Don't like the car! Where's my mummy?!* and, *Watch 'Paw'trol'* (Paw Patrol) were some of the things you screamed in protest from your car seat.

Most of what we ask you to do is met with a response of *don't want to do!* You have certainly started to develop your independence!

The accidents continue to roll as you earnt yourself a bruised eye after tripping up and falling into the radiator!

Mummy is making attempts at trying to make your hair look slightly presentable, cutting bits of it at a time.

Your bedtime story was the *'Jim-Jim'* (Gingerbread) *Man* for the third night in a row.

**22nd April 2020**
You have started entertaining yourself in your bedroom when you wake up which is a welcome change to coming straight downstairs at 6.45am and demanding *Paw Patrol* or *The Land Before Time* on the television!

We are having to keep a lid on your bossiness and defiance otherwise you really would end up ruling the house – *No! Do it that way! OK?!*

We witnessed the most amazing thing on our daily walk. Climbing the hill we spotted a sheep in a field looking more than uncomfortable. Close by, a farmer told us that the lamb next to it was ten minutes old. He then crouched down, rolled up his sleeve and helped the sheep give birth to another lamb. You imaginatively named the newborn *Little Lamb*.

Saif and Kaiser spoiled you again with some chocolates and an ice cream whilst you played football with me in the garden.

We were told by the Government that we are now 'at the peak' of the Covid-19 outbreak and 18,100 people have now died in UK hospitals. We will have to wait and see whether that's the case.

### 23rd April 2020

*Elbows!* – a reference to the safest way of greeting someone in the midst of a pandemic – was all you said to me as I walked out of the front door to work!

You tackled the 'dusty bank' – a relatively steep embankment at the side of the path round the back of the estate – on your own in my absence. *That's fun!* you declared after managing to hold your balance running down!

Last week, we noticed that the lack of socialisation was leading to you being wary of others. You now appear to have shaken this off, telling anyone you encounter what you have been doing on your walk. On returning, you kindly told a lady near the house that you were *going for a poo behind Daddy's car!*

It is also apparent that you will wee on demand for *Paw Patrol* stickers. This led to you doing seven in an hour!

Soon after you were put to bed it was time for another Thursday-night clap for the NHS workers on the front doorstep. People brought pots and pans and banged them with wooden spoons. It is a rare form of isolated group socialisation, both heart-warming and emotional at the same time.

### 24th April 2020
You are very good at setting the table for breakfast – *Mat, bowl, spoon, milk, Cheerios!*

Clearing away, though, is another matter. Your third-person retort to Mummy asking you to tidy up was, *Noah's going in the front room… Mummy do it!* Your ability to speak in full sentences now means that you can fluently answer back!

It passed 20°C for the first time in lockdown so we got the paddling pool out in the garden. All was going well until someone set fireworks off in the middle of spring and you decided that you no longer liked pyrotechnics!

### 25th April 2020
It was a Saturday – our fifth weekend in lockdown. There was talk in the news about how we will possibly be able to mix with two other households soon as the Government ponders how to ease us back to normality.

You wanted to play football with Mrs Arain, asking her to kick the ball back over the fence after you had thrown it to her. Later in the day you gave her a picture you had done with felt-tip pens and stickers.

Almost 21,000 people have now died from Covid-19 in UK hospitals. These would fill Manchester Arena.

### 26th April 2020
The nice weather continued and we enjoyed our third day of sunshine in succession.

You applied your own sun cream and declared that you liked the smell, before deciding to taste a sample off your hand!

On our walk you were disappointed to discover that the *wobbedy* flag at the top of hill had been fixed with tarmac. You were beset by clumsiness and must have fallen over about fifteen times whilst we were out. At the street corner before home you toppled over, grazing your nose and forehead.

Dave, our next-door neighbour, gave you some newts in a jar from his pond. Mummy wrongly told you that a newt follows a tadpole in the life cycle of a frog!

One of your tropical fish died today. Not that you noticed.

### 27th April 2020

As you checked out your reflection in the mirror you whined, *Don't want a sore nose!*

Since seeing a lamb being born, stopping off to look at the sheep has become a daily occurrence. Today, you treated them to your own rendition of 'Baa, Baa, Black Sheep'.

Today's Covid-19 deaths in hospitals totalled 360, which is the lowest daily increase since the end of March.

### 28th April 2020

Spring is well underway and the plants, flowers and trees are blooming. You are finding out which ones sting and which ones prickle. You managed to get several small thorns stuck in your fingers and the palm of your hand so you asked me to hold your '*tum*' (thumb), as opposed to your hand, on our daily walk.

For the majority of the afternoon you did things you should not have been doing and behaved like a general nuisance.

Video calls have become a bit tedious, with no social activities to report on, and you have started to shout *bye!* prematurely at whoever it is you are talking to. This is usually followed by you pointing your elbow at the screen and asking for a *Wuhan kiss.*

### 29th April 2020

Miraculously, it has taken this long for us to have a rainy day in lockdown. Grandad Col came to drop some things off so you spent time playing football at a 'social distance' with him in the garden.

Eleven horses had been released into one of the fields we usually walk through. They were a bit anxious and edgy so we decided to take a slight diversion. You still wanted to greet them and shouted, *Hello!* from afar.

I put my wellies on for a change, which you were happy about because it meant you had a new puddle-splashing partner.

Afternoons through the week can become difficult when we are trying to work. You are clearly tired but fight against it because you want to be busy.

You picked the scab that has formed on your nose throughout the day, telling us *don't want it*, and asking us to *make it go away!*

Before bed you hopped around the floor pretending to be a frog whilst speaking to Great-Grandad Mike, Great-Nan Ann, Grandad Ste, Sharon, Stevie and Simon on a family video call.

Until now, the Government has only released the numbers of people who have died from Covid-19 in hospital. Today, we learnt the full extent of deaths in hospitals, care homes and the community. It stands at a grim 26,097.

**30<sup>th</sup> April 2020**

Today would have been Great-Grandad Alan's ninetieth birthday.

Sitting on the couch watching television before breakfast, as we tried to get a head-start with our jobs on the laptops, you demanded, *Mummy! Daddy! No working! OK?!* It was not the first time during lockdown where you expressed your dissatisfaction at us having to work.

Your caterpillar metamorphosis set arrived in the post and you put the box of baby caterpillars next to your tropical fish tank.

Regrettably, Mummy and I are overusing the television to keep you busy whilst we work. I took you for a break from screen time, playing football outside in the pouring rain. You told me off for flicking the ball over the fence. *Kick the ball on the grass*, you instructed, pointing to the lawn.

I was on my way back from completing the weekly shop at the time of the 8pm clap for the NHS so beeped my horn at people stood at their doors on the way back up the hill.

The Government announced the five tests for adjusting the strict lockdown rules:

The NHS must be able to provide treatment and care all over the UK.

Daily deaths must continue to fall.

Proof that the rate of infection, known as the R, is decreasing to manageable levels.

Testing and Personal Protective Equipment (PPE), such as face masks and gloves, must be widely available.

Confidence that any adjustments to the current measures will not risk a second peak of Covid-19 infections that would once again overwhelm the NHS.

**1st May 2020**
This is now the third calendar month we have been in isolation. It is going to be another week before we learn from the Government what the first step out of it is going to look like.

Even though all the days seem the same, Fridays tend to be a touch more relaxed as Mummy and I have completed a lot of the work we need to do for the week.

You enjoy leaving bread in the garden for the *birdies* but do not like the excess poo this leaves on our conservatory roof and wooden sleepers in the garden.

You are a thoughtful, helpful little boy and have started to assist Mummy and I over the stiles on our walks.

After telling us you want to see another deer throughout April we eventually saw one today... not before emptying your wellies with half a litre of water after jumping in the stream!

**2nd May 2020**
The fact that Mummy and I wanted a lie-in led to a meltdown of epic proportions! You were so aggrieved that you threw a flip-flop at me once I made it downstairs into the kitchen!

The potty-training is progressing well, probably because you get a sticker and a chocolate after every visit. Today was actually the first day since starting training that you did not wet yourself. We were so proud!

Due to the lack of socialisation that isolation inevitably brings you have again started to become wary and apprehensive. You do not like the rare sight of an aeroplane flying overhead, you cover your eyes when cars drive past on our walks and you do not like interaction with strangers.

We hid a dinosaur egg for you near the 'dusty bank' when we were out and you were very excited to take this home and show your teddies!

You had a daytime nap for the first time in almost a week which meant you were not tired at bedtime. This led to you coming downstairs with us whilst we were on a video call doing a quiz with friends. Lockdown has meant people have opened their imagination when spending time with one another online and such things go some way towards raising morale.

### 3rd May 2020

After you were born, I somehow managed to have five weeks off work. This is now the longest continuous period of time that I have ever spent with you.

You scratched your hand on our walk and thought that this could be cured with a dock leaf!

An important part of potty-training is helping you improve your aim when stood up. Daddy advised you to *shake it*, so you did not dribble after your pee stream had ceased. This led to you picking up your potty and swirling it around!

When playing football you do not want to take a touch before passing, or kick it with your weaker right foot – *No! Kick it with left foot!* you shout!

**4<sup>th</sup> May 2020**
The day started with you trying to dictate where everyone was allowed to sit in the front room.

We walked down through the dell after lunch to find the *Gruffalo's cave*. When you saw the stream your imagination transported you to the wilds of Africa and you asked Mummy, *Where's the hippos?*

You are getting good at playing with your *Paw Patrol* characters on your own, creating problems for the pups to rescue one another from whilst singing your own version of the theme track.

Rumours in the press suggest that the Government will announce the lockdown exit strategy on Sunday 10<sup>th</sup> May.

**5<sup>th</sup> May 2020**
The dinosaur egg you found a few days ago hatched this morning and out popped a stegosaurus which you named *Baby*.

After enduring six weeks of our intensive potty-training programme you finally did a poo in the little, white well and earnt yourself a 'Kinder Egg'.

You went nappyless on the walk and had a wee in the stream, failing to be put off by a nosey horse that came for a look at what you were doing!

We saw hundreds of tadpoles in the pond and then

you climbed up a steep bank – *a mountain* – and played 'tig' with me.

Your attachment to your *Paw Patrol* figures is admirable. You like them so much that you want them to watch you shower and get in bed with you!

### 6th May 2020

This morning you told us that you loved your teddies (Chase, Gruffalo, Monkey and Tiger) and your blanket *more than Mummy and Daddy*!

Lockdown has led to an increase in alcohol consumption for many households and ours is no different. You and Mummy had to go to Auntie Stevie's to fill her bottle bin up with our empties.

Initially, you were a bit freaked out by the sight of number two's in the potty. Now you like to describe them and, apparently, one you did today *looked like a snail!*

Before bed you helped Mummy and Daddy mark out our plans for an extension to the back of our house with chalk on the flags. You soon lost interest in the task at hand and defaced the BBQ, sleepers and windows instead!

### 7th May 2020

Today you went to Grandma and Grandad's for the first time since 21st March. Grandad came to drop a thermometer off for your fish tank and we let you go back with him. Darcie had been for a few hours the day before so we let you do the same.

It was a decision that was made after much discussion between Mummy and I about what was best. Admittedly it was against lockdown restrictions but we felt that the risk was low. You enjoyed playing in the football nets with Grandad in his garden. He had bought these for you more than seven weeks ago and you had yet to use them.

You fell asleep in the car on the way back home so it was the first day since lockdown began that you did not go for a walk.

We still have three days to wait until we know how the relaxation measures will change lockdown, if at all.

The virus claimed the lives of 539 people today bringing the total number of deaths to 30,615.

**8th May 2020**
Your little legs are now able to walk up to two and a half miles. Grandma and Grandad joined us today, maintaining a social distance. You claimed to have found Makka Pakka's, from *In the Night Garden*, stones in the dell.

We went for a drive and you fell asleep less than a mile into the trip. We called at Great-Nana Mave's to collect some eggs and she showed you off to her neighbours. We then dropped some of your paintings off for Nana Roz, James, Grandad Ste and Sharon.

It was a Friday Bank Holiday, not that it makes much difference in lockdown, due to Victory in Europe (VE) Day. This marked the seventy-fifth anniversary of the end of World War Two. On the way home we saw lots of people having 'socially distant' street parties and houses were decorated with Union Jack flags and banners.

At home we had a water fight in the garden. You soon mastered how to use your water tube and took great delight in soaking Mummy and Daddy.

As I caught up with writing this book you sat wrapped

in a towel in the garden having just got out of your paddling pool – *What you doing, Daddy? My willy hurts!*

Well, that's what happens, Little Man, when you continuously pull on it!

### 9th May 2020

Nothing is stronger than a child who does not want to get in their car seat! That was certainly the case with you before we drove up to the reservoirs for a walk. We enjoyed the hottest day of lockdown so far as we walked around the middle reservoir. You were convinced that there were sharks in the water that were going to eat the geese!

### 10th May 2020

You can get a bit lazy now that you are not wearing a nappy but you definitely pushed your luck when you intentionally did a wee on the kitchen floor. *That's not rude!* you insisted. I think you will find it is, Little Man!

Boris Johnson addressed the nation at 7pm. He stressed, 'Now is not the time for lockdown to end.' However, from tomorrow, people who cannot work from home can go to their workplace.

From Wednesday next week people can exercise and play sports outdoors as long as it is with members of their own household.

The prime minister announced that had the country not gone into lockdown at least half a million people would have lost their lives. Despite the strict restrictions that have been imposed, 31,855 people have now died in the UK.

Chapter 4

# EASING LOCKDOWN (PHASE ONE)

**11th May 2020**

The Government's slogan of 'Stay at home, protect the NHS, save lives' has been changed to 'Stay alert, control the virus, save lives'. It received a fair amount of criticism. Especially since it is rather difficult to 'stay alert' to something that is only 120 nanometres in diameter!

This phase now means that non-essential workers can return to work. You can meet with one other person outside your household and travel to the beach to socialise.

Not much has changed in our household but Mummy may have to go back into work on 1st June.

Your new favourite phrase is *that's funny!* and you like playing your own game of 'What time is it Mr Wolf?' *Stop! Go!* you quickly shout intermittently.

Whilst your afternoon nap is a welcome break in terms of being able to get on with our work, it is counterproductive when it comes to you going to sleep on time at night. Well past bedtime, you regularly checked on us from the landing and took it upon yourself to explore the other rooms upstairs.

It was in the news that professional sport may resume on 1$^{st}$ June from behind closed doors.

### 12$^{th}$ May 2020 – Fiftieth Day in Lockdown
Dr Noah likes to give us a daily medical with his new doctor's set! To our relief, the only health issue you diagnosed was *worms* in our ears and throat!

You spent the afternoon with Grandma, Grandad and Darcie. You were very excited to tell me what you had been up to when I got home from work.

Before bed you recorded a birthday message for Darcie, whose birthday is tomorrow, holding your wooden cake set. You picked a candle up that had dropped on the floor and pretended to blow it out! Funny!

### 13$^{th}$ May 2020
Darcie was two years old today so we sang 'Happy birthday!' to her over a video call.

Grandma and Grandad picked you up before lunch. Before you left Mummy made you pick up the jigsaw pieces you had thrown around the front room in temper!

You had a look at the bird box Grandad had made – *Want to see where the birdies live!*

We went to Liam, Emma and Darcie's house for tea. Uncle Kyle, Auntie Alice and Alice's sister Amy were also there 'social distancing' in the garden with Grandma and Grandad.

You liked playing with Darcie's doll's house, helped Darcie blow out the candles on her birthday cake, and then ate three slices of it!

We pushed you home in your pram and you insisted on me pushing you *faster*, which led to me running most of the way!

**14<sup>th</sup> May 2020**
*What time is it?* is your new favourite question even though you have no concept of how clocks work.

You enjoyed joining in Mummy's video call with her class, roaring with your favourite dinosaur and singing the songs louder than her children!

I walked you in your pram to collect my car from near Darcie's house. You missed the usual rural experience, as we walked through the housing estate, asking to see the various animals we usually see on our walks.

Several moments today kind of epitomised your innocence as a bright, two-year-old boy. First, you brought one of Mummy's sanitary products from the bathroom and asked if it was chocolate.

Stevie and Simon stayed for a short while in the garden after dropping some sunflower seeds off for you. On their way out, not wanting them to go, you blocked their exit via the gate. This caused us all to choke with emotion. It was very difficult to explain to you what 'happy tears' were.

You were still awake for the 8pm clap which has become a national ritual. *What's that noise? Where's everyone clapping gone? Where's NHS?*

Bless you, Little Man!

## 15th May 2020

Mummy and I were really busy with work so you went to Grandma and Grandad's for a few hours. Whilst against lockdown restrictions, it certainly alleviates the pressure of trying to complete our day jobs whilst caring for you.

You went for a walk through the valley and when you came home you told us all about the *cow poo* you had seen. Apparently, it was horse manure on the road and actual cows in the field and you had become a bit mixed up when recalling the events.

A pattern is emerging where you wet yourself on purpose through defiance. I told you that your potty-training was 'going backwards', which you responded to by moonwalking across the kitchen!

You are now confident enough to walk round to the neighbours to ask for your ball back when you have kicked it over the fence.

## 16th May 2020

I played golf in the morning with Grandad Col, the first time we had both picked up a club since 21st March. The Government's ruling is that you are allowed to participate in sport with one other person outside of your household as long as you observe social distancing.

Nana Roz and James called after lunch to drop off some Easter eggs and clothes. We then went for a walk around the back of the solitary windmill on the hill. There was a little boy at the alpacas and he gave you some carrots to feed them.

The Bundesliga, German football's premier division, started back up again. Live sport has been non-existent since the start of lockdown so I wanted to watch it. The problem with this was you did not want to go to sleep and, given you have had control of the television for the best part of eight weeks, would not part with the remote!

### 17th May 2020
The caterpillars have now grown *big and fat* and made themselves cocoons. In a week or so you should have five butterflies to release!

We went for a two and half mile walk with Stevie and Simon and you were desperate to show them all your favourite things from the walks we have done. Stevie had a sleep when she got home. You did not!

We called at Grandma and Grandad's to pick up some tea Grandma had made for us. On the way home we stopped at Liam and Emma's to collect a gardening fork. Darcie was so happy to see you and so upset when we left after a few minutes. *My 'Woah'!* (Noah) she screamed as we all got back in the car.

### 18th May 2020
You woke up at 5am crying because of a 'devastating' dream. *Daddy! Don't eat my crisps!* you wailed. Thankfully, the traumatic experience did not stop you falling back asleep!

We are now into our ninth week of working from home and it is not getting any easier.

Nursery contacted us to ask if you will be going back on 1st June. If Mummy has to go back to work on the same day then we will have no choice but to send you in. The good thing is that you will probably be going to the same one as Darcie after circumstances dictated that you had to attend separate ones last September. This was because Liam and Emma pass a different one on their way to work.

On the walk you insisted that you had to lead from the front and declared you were taking us to see the pigs. Pigs are about the only farm animal we have yet to see in lockdown! We were not sure where you thought you were going!

160 people died from Covid-19 today, the lowest total since the start of lockdown, bringing the total number of deaths to 34,796. So much devastation for so many families which we have luckily managed to escape ourselves.

### 19th May 2020

Mummy took you to Grandma and Grandad's in the morning where you stayed for a few hours. On the way you said that you wanted Nana Roz, James, Stevie, Simon, Grandad Ste, Sharron and the rest of the family to go too.

When you got home you proudly informed us that you had kicked a ball in Darcie's face! Grandma let us know that Darcie was unhurt but your honesty was admirable all the same!

You went for a walk with me to allow Mummy to continue working and found a 1p coin, dated 1936. So pleased you were at finding something 84 years old that you threw it in a bush!

Getting you out of the bath is a tough task as you do not want the water to disappear. Once it is all gone you lie on your front, tuck your knees into your chest and swear you are a frog!

You did not want to put a nappy on for bed and protested as I pinned you down! You chuckled heartily as

Mummy managed to get one round your ankles and knees and pulled it up to your waist!

**21st May 2020**
After an early 5.45am rise for you, your conversation with me went like this:
*Where you going, Daddy?*
'I'm going to work to get a promotion, Little Man'.
*No… getting ocean?!*
Later in the day:
'Who's birthday is it on Sunday, Noah?'
*Grandad Col's!*
'How old is he?'
*Two!* was your reply.
'No! He's not two! He's sixty!'
*Not sixty! It's Friday!*
And in the bath:
*Need a wee!*
Mummy told you to aim for the plug hole.
*No, Mummy! Not a hole! Not a bumble bee's house* (a reference to seeing bees travel to and from a hole in a mound of mud on one walk during lockdown)… *it is a plug!*

So, I got my promotion and I am now classed as experienced in my profession.

Mummy was informed that the earliest she will be returning to work in the classroom will be 15th June. We are both undecided about when will be best to allow you to return to nursery.

**22nd May 2020**
I went to work so you and Mummy enjoyed a walk as a

duo. It was a windy day and you held on to Mummy's hand tightly to stop her from blowing away!

We all played cricket in the garden whilst cooking on the BBQ. Mummy caught and bowled you twice but your stubbornness meant you refused to let either of us bat.

You fell asleep at the table after your tea so I carried you to bed. Mummy putting a nappy on you woke you up and you demanded to wear underpants for bed. Conceding to a toddler is sometimes easier than the fight so we put the potty in your room. This could be fun!

**23rd May 2020**
Wahey! You slept in your underpants all night and did not wet them! Throughout lockdown, we are witnessing your evolution from a toddler into a little boy! When I got home from golf you excitedly showed me that two of your cocoons were now butterflies!

In the afternoon you went to the park with Grandma and Grandad. You were more interested in throwing stones in the lake then you were in looking at the ducks and geese on it.

With you out of the house, Mummy and I relished the opportunity to watch a football match from the Bundesliga – Borussia Möenchengladbach (1) vs Bayer Leverkusen (3).

We all danced in the kitchen after tea. 'Lion Sleeps Tonight' from *The Lion King* and Craig David's 'Walking Away' are currently your favourite non-children's tunes!

**24th May 2020**
'Who's your best friend, Noah?'
*Grandad!*

Given today is Grandad Col's sixtieth birthday, we will let you off! Grandma and Grandad were supposed to be having a joint sixtieth birthday party today at a local restaurant but large gatherings are not permitted due to lockdown. Instead, they had a small 'socially distant' gathering in their spacious garden.

**25$^{th}$ May 2020**
The weather was even nicer today so I got carried away at the butcher's and we had a BBQ at home. The nice weather throughout lockdown has offered some welcome relief to people up and down the country.

We released the five butterflies we had watched grow from tiny caterpillars. You loved putting them on your hands before they flew away *high in the sky*.

**26$^{th}$ May 2020**
You woke up with a limp and told us that you had stood on a screw. There was no clear evidence of any injury.

It is Mummy's half-term so she took you to the park where you surprisingly bumped into Grandma, Grandad and Darcie! You were then 'mauled' by a Shih Tzu puppy, who dived after the teddy you dropped when you fell over.

Before you were born Mummy and I attended some classes with other expectant parents to learn how to care for you as a newborn baby. This afternoon you painted a pottery gingerbread man on a video call with Mummy, the other mummies who attended the classes and their children. It is great how you all still keep in touch.

**27th May 2020**

If we had not been in lockdown we would have been going to St Andrew's in Scotland with Grandma and Grandad. I was meant to take Grandad to play golf on the famous Old Course as part of his sixtieth birthday present.

As a result, I am off work until 1st June so we are just going to have a 'holiday' at home.

Mummy was in work so you came to Dunsop Bridge with me, Grandma, Grandad and Darcie. We had a picnic on the green and you enjoyed throwing pebbles into the river. It was difficult getting you to stick to your overarm throw, as opposed to your underarm version where your release point varies from throw to throw!

You were not tired at bedtime and you have now developed the stalling tactic of climbing out of bed and demanding us to *cover* (me) *up!* from the top of the stairs. That, and singing, *Glory! Glory! Man United!* until 9.45pm!

**28th May 2020**

Mummy and I took you and Darcie to the highest beach in England at Gaddings Dam. It was a very steep climb for two toddlers so we stopped twice on the ascent to tuck into our picnic.

At the top, there were people swimming in the disused reservoir, where swimmers train for triathlons, and enjoying disposable BBQs. It was busy but you could tell people were wary of getting close to others who were not with them. You and Darcie both loved paddling in the water.

On the way down, you were a combination of tired, hot and giddy and kept running off to hide behind boulders.

Back home you and Darcie played with water in the

garden. You both refused to wear any clothes because it was so hot.

The English Premier League is set to resume from behind closed doors on 17th June.

**29th May 2020**
We went for a drive to Formby Beach and had another picnic. Mummy and I had to hide the cocktail sausages from you because that is all you wanted to eat!

You walked with me across the sand to the sea which was quite far out. The vast amount of lugworm casts in the sand disturbed you somewhat. *Wiggle wiggle worms*, you anxiously pointed. The possibility that they could also be in the water prevented you from going into the sea!

We have booked to go to Cornwall in August and hope that the lockdown restrictions will have been relaxed as we are meant to be staying in a house with Grandma, Grandad, Liam, Emma and Darcie.

**30th May 2020**
After breakfast Mummy took you to see Great-Nana Anne with Auntie Stevie so that Great-Grandad Mike could go out for a ride on his motorbike.

You introduced her to all your *Paw Patrol* figures and played Humpty Dumpty, knocking her garden ornaments off the wall.

When Great-Grandad Mike returned the plan was for you to sit on his motorbike but you were scared of him in his leathers!

You have started to call people *silly* but do not understand the context. Great-Nana Anne is struggling with her memory and she ate Great-Grandad Mike's piece of cake. This led to you calling Grandad *silly*.

You made their day as they have not seen you since before the country was plunged into lockdown.

## 31st May 2020

The morning was spent gardening and you were quite the little helper. When the lawnmower broke down you went inside and asked Mummy for some *ketchup* to get it started again. It is certainly a mystery where your mind takes you at times!

Mummy and I felt emotional walking you past the horses, tadpoles and alpacas. Our walks will not be as frequent for the time being as you are returning to nursery tomorrow.

The last few weeks have begun to bring a slight sense of normality back to us as a family. Although we should not really have done, we took the decision to see a small number of close family and friends. In doing so, we have created happy memories during what has been a hugely difficult time.

From tomorrow, you will be going back to nursery for three days a week. Your nursery is still closed so you will be going to a different one within the same company.

Some schools are opening their doors to certain year groups tomorrow, although Mummy's school will not be opening until at least 15th June.

In the next phase of lockdown-easing the Government have decided to allow us to socialise with up to five people from different households. This means that groups of six can spend time together as long as they are outside and social distancing is observed.

We will not be spending as much time with you over the next few weeks so this book may not continue to follow an almost-daily account of your life.

More than two months since the start of lockdown, 39,045 people have lost their lives to Covid-19. The concern is that if lockdown is lifted too soon there could be a 'spike' in infections and tougher measures could return. This has already happened in Germany. The journey through the unknown continues for us all.

Chapter 5

# EASING LOCKDOWN (PHASE TWO)

**1st June 2020**
I had to go into work so Mummy was left with the unenvious task of taking you to nursery for the first time in ten weeks. This was very tough. As Mummy tried to hand you over to the nursery staff you clung to her leg, tears streaming down your face, heartbroken. We had made the decision for you to return based on wanting you to socialise with little boys and girls of your own age. And anyway, we knew how much you loved going before the start of the pandemic.

Thankfully, you soon settled and the emotion of the morning meant you had a long nap in the afternoon.

You were so excited to see Mummy when she picked you up, telling her all about your day. You were delighted that a train track ran behind the back of your temporary nursery!

When I got home you gave me a big hug and told me that you were looking forward to going to nursery again tomorrow!

## 2nd June 2020

You asked me to take you to nursery this morning. When you got to the door, despite singing joyfully to the irritating Pinkfong album in the car, you were equally adamant that you did not want to part with me for your day in education! Again, you had a great day and emerged from the door at home time filthy!

The three of us went to Great-Nana Mave's house for a 'socially distant' chippy on her drive with Nana Roz, James, Stevie and Simon. You charmed Great-Nana Mave's neighbours with your cheeky personality and came home with a bag of treats off them.

You are not adapting too well to the increasingly lighter nights and have developed some stalling tactics when we try and put you to bed. Tonight's was to refuse to pull your underpants down to do your bedtime wee on your potty!

## 3rd June 2020

Nana Roz woke up with symptoms of Covid-19, a headache and aches and pains all over her body. She had to go to hospital for a test and the results can take up to three days to come back. As we were in close proximity to her yesterday we are now at risk of carrying Covid-19 or becoming ill from the virus ourselves. You are at a lower risk because children have not been affected as much by the coronavirus.

As such, I had to come home from work in case I had

picked up the virus from Nana Roz. This was even though we were all outside and stayed more than two metres away from one another.

We now need to self-isolate until Nana Roz gets her test results back. If it is positive then we will not be able to leave our house until 17th June.

This is the first time in lockdown that we have had tangible concern that family members may have contracted Covid-19. This is especially the case for Nana Mave and Auntie Stevie, who are part of the more vulnerable sections of society due to age and health conditions respectively.

**4th June 2020**
*Back to square one*, I had you saying all day. That is what it felt like as we had to work from home. After two emotional days of going back to nursery, you are at home with us once again!

Nana Roz said that she was feeling a bit better, despite the constant aching. She did not feel as ill as the time she thought she had contracted Covid-19 off James earlier in lockdown. There is no news on whether the test she took yesterday is positive or not.

We went for a walk before our tea, washing our hands first and taking a route where we did not have to touch anything. It is amazing how green everything has turned since the end of March when we came into lockdown.

**5th June 2020**
Today, you turned two and a half years old!

*It is morning time!* you audibly announced as you walked down the stairs.

Nana Roz's Covid-19 test came back negative which means we are back to how we were a few days ago. There is great relief as we do not have to worry about anyone else who was there for the chippy tea on Nana Mave's drive.

Even though we had been careful not to get close to one another, and constantly sanitised our hands, a paranoia crept in as we reflected on such a small window of socialisation.

You are oblivious to such painful, emotional realities of living in lockdown. What was real to you, however, was biting your thumb whilst eating at both lunch and teatime! Ouch!

## 6th June 2020

Whilst I was at golf, you spent the morning reading books with Mummy. Your memory is fantastic and you have a genuine love of children's literature. You are almost able to fully recount the story of *The Snail and the Whale*.

In the afternoon we went to Grandma and Grandad's and spent time in the garden. You like being a goalkeeper but tend to dive over most of the shots you face.

You said that the meatballs we had for tea were *too spicy*. Grandad tried to encourage you to eat your spaghetti by referring to them as 'wiggly worms'. This did not have the desired effect as you soon remembered the worm casts from the beach!

## 7th June 2020

Fifty-five people died of Covid-19 today. This was the first time the total had been below one hundred since the start of lockdown. 40,597 people's lives have now been taken by the virus in the UK.

## 8th June 2020

Back to nursery! Despite your small protest at home you were happy to walk to the door yourself and there were no tears. Your own nursery is scheduled to reopen on 22nd June.

You were a monkey all day, perhaps a sign that you were becoming comfortable in the environment. After lunch, staff became worried that you had been in the toilet on your own for a while. On inspection, it was because you had taken a doll with you and spent some time washing her in the sink!

It is Uncle Kyle's thirtieth birthday next week so we tried to get you to sing some United songs for him on a video message. Instead of the new Bruno Fernandes song you gave him a rendition of 'Baby Shark!'.

Maybe we'll try again tomorrow!

## 9th June 2020

When lockdown started you were a toddler who still wore nappies and liked to drink his milk from a Tommee Tippee bottle. Now, you are a little boy who manages to keep his underpants dry through the night and no longer enjoys his morning milk through a teat! The bottle has gone and it feels as though you are no longer a baby!

The nursery staff continue to endure your cheeky nature. Today, you laughed at the manager whilst she was telling you off!

## 11th June 2020

When Mummy and I were two years old we did not have a choice about what we watched on television. As we grew older we had to wait, sometimes as long as a week, for our favourite programmes to come on television. In 2020, you are demanding which specific *Paw Patrol* episode you want on Netflix. *Volcano Paw'trol! Fireworks Paw'trol!* This is a very difficult need to meet, especially since there are 156 episodes to scroll through!

I picked you up from nursery and the staff did not have to tell me you had been pushing children over in the garden because you proudly owned up to it immediately! You are certainly not a naughty boy but, annoyingly, staff do like to highlight when you have been up to mischief! I suppose it is their job.

### 12th June 2020

Today should have marked the start of more than four weeks of international football. The first game of UEFA Euro 2020 was set to take place between Italy and Turkey in Rome, Italy. So far, there have been 34,167 Covid-19 deaths in Italy so it was certainly a wise decision to postpone the competition.

Nana Roz has reluctantly made the choice to suspend caring for you on a Friday. This is because there are still lots of people with Covid-19 on the ward she works on. The NHS is drowning under the weight of the pandemic with not enough beds to care for those who have contracted the virus.

A lady who works with Mummy has got some baby rabbits so we have decided to take two off her for you as pets. One is called Marble, due to the pattern of his fur, but the other has not got a name yet.

### 13th June 2020

Dates come and go where social events would have otherwise taken place had it not been for the pandemic.

Last Saturday should have been Nana Roz's hen party. Today, I was supposed to go and watch England play cricket against the West Indies in a Test match at Edgbaston, Birmingham.

You went to your friend Eric's farm with Mummy and loved playing in the mud. You were not too keen on the donkey's loud hee-hawing!

We are now ready for the pending arrival of our two rabbits after constructing their wooden hutch in the garden. We were hoping to get the rabbits today but we are having to wait until next Saturday. Coincidentally, this is the same day another pet will be welcomed into the family as Stevie and Simon are getting a puppy. There has been a huge rise in the purchase of pets during lockdown, with the new-found companionship supporting people's mental health.

I tried to teach you to catch a big, soft ball in the garden. You kind of misunderstood my tip to 'keep your eye on the ball' because each time you threw it back you advised me to *catch my eyes!*

Today, you had your first visit to the ice-cream van which has started doing the rounds on our street. It is now very difficult to curb your curiosity when its chime becomes audible. You had a *pink one* (strawberry) with a flake and raspberry sauce.

### 15th June 2020

Mummy went back to school for the first time since 20th March. When she got there, the parents of seven children who she had expected to be present had changed their minds. This was due to pressure from people in the community who did not feel as though it was right for schools to reopen in the middle of a pandemic.

Non-essential shops opened as well for the first time today. There are restrictions on how many customers can enter at one time and you are only allowed to touch what you are going to buy. In some ways, it feels as though we are slowly moving back to normal.

I had to go to Ludlow, Shropshire, with work. The service stations were quiet, with one-way systems in place to keep people away from one another. Most of the shops in the town centre were still shut.

On the way home I inadvertently broke lockdown rules. I stopped for something to eat in Wrexham, completely forgetting that I should not have entered Wales as a non-resident!

### 17th June 2020

The English Premier League resumed after a one hundred-day absence. Aston Villa and Sheffield United drew 0–0 behind closed doors. A minute's silence was held to remember the lives of people claimed by Covid-19. Players wore heart-shaped badges on their kits to pay tribute to NHS workers.

On 25th May, a black man named George Floyd was killed in the United States of America by a white police officer. This led to race protests around the world. Players from both sides took a knee before the game in a stand against racism and other forms of discrimination. The Premier League confirmed that players would wear 'Black

Lives Matter' on the back of their shirts for the final twelve rounds of games following the resumption of the league.

The remaining ninety-two games will be played before the last round of matches on 26th July. Players and staff have been tested for Covid-19 twice a week for the last eight weeks and this will continue moving forwards. So far, there have been sixteen positive results from 8,687 tests.

The stalling tactics at bedtime continued as you claimed that you wanted to watch the thunder and lightning outside. I suppose it would be worse if you were scared of it!

**18th June 2020**

Instead of coming downstairs and demanding milk and *Paw'trol* on the television you sat in the kitchen quietly playing with your cars whilst I made you a crumpet. The mornings are quieter now that your protests about going to nursery have died down. Normality has resumed in the sense that you are loving going again.

When you came home Mummy and I came up with a phrase to try and combat the 'terrible twos' phase you are currently in: 'Listen with your ears and then there's no tears'.

With your quest for independence, your defiance and tantrums can be challenging. We find it very difficult to hold our laughs in at some of your inexplicable behaviour!

**19th June 2020**

Grandma took you and Darcie to Carol's farm. Carol is someone else who has missed you during lockdown, having been accustomed to seeing you every week at the park. You and Darcie loved looking at the animals and feeding Tilly, the baby goat, milk from a bottle.

Auntie Stevie required an emergency operation in hospital today. She was lucky the operation went ahead as it was vital she had the treatment. Lots of other people have had operations cancelled due to the pandemic as the NHS continues to struggle to cope with the demand created by Covid-19. At least when the operation was finished she got to go home to an eight-week old springer spaniel named Harley.

United played their first game following the suspension of the Premier League, drawing 1–1 away at Tottenham Hotspur. There were no fans in the stadium but crowd noise was played through people's televisions. It was all very surreal and the tempo and pace of the game was certainly not the same as it might have been in front of a capacity crowd.

**20th June 2020**
In the morning you went for a walk with Mummy and her friend Shelley. You tripped up near a pond and almost ended up with your face in the water.

When I got back from golf you helped Mummy and I prepare the rabbit hutch with a huge bag of sawdust. Marble, a female, and a white male rabbit the moved into our home. You were so gentle with them and really enjoyed stroking them on your knee. After a bit of consultation, Mummy and I decided to name the white rabbit Quartz. We supposed it complemented Marble, although they do sound like the name of a kitchen worktop company!

Welcoming two new pets into the home was a draining

affair for you. This culminated in you falling asleep in your rice pudding at 5.50pm!

**21st June 2020**
Father's Day. *Happy Farmer's Day!* you wished me, joyfully.

We met Stevie and Simon's puppy Harley for the first time! You were both getting along so well until you accidentally flung a tennis ball in her face!

Grandad Ste and Sharron did not see much of you because you fell asleep on the way to their house and then stayed asleep for the duration of time we were there!

I decided that we should go to Hebden Bridge as their restaurants, bars and cafés were serving takeaway food and drink. We ate in the square and Mummy and I bought a beer from a bar for the first time in twelve weeks. You enjoyed a *dough-nup* (doughnut) from the bakery and then fed the ducks.

We went to Grandma and Grandad's for tea and travelled home in a taxi for the first time since lockdown began.

**22nd June 2020**
Your own nursery opened and the change in environment set you back as you clung to Mummy's leg at the door once more.

After yesterday's introduction you wanted to go and see Harley again. She remembered you though and was too scared to come near you!

After a two-hour nap at nursery, bedtime came too early for you. You are now wanting at least five United songs, as well as a story, before you will entertain the idea of going to sleep!

**23rd June 2020**
It was announced that sections of the hospitality industry – restaurants, cinemas, theatres and pubs – will open on 4th July. Social distancing will halve from two metres to one metre if it cannot be avoided. A glint of hope, perhaps.

Social distancing is not a principle that you currently abide by at nursery as you told me that you had been *kissing girls* today!

You are bonding with Marble and Quartz, cuddling them and saying *Aww* as you rest your head softly on their bodies.

Nana Roz's cat Pudsey was put to sleep today. She was nineteen and Mummy had known her since she was fifteen years old herself.

**24th June 2020**
Grandma Buckley's sixtieth birthday. You have now moved away from thinking that every time someone celebrates a birthday they are turning two like you. Unfortunately for Grandma, you said she was seventy!

The hottest day of the year, a sweltering 29°C. Grandma's friend allowed us to socialise at the back of her restaurant and you played with bubbles on the bowling green.

United beat Sheffield United 3–0 at Old Trafford. Anthony Martial scored our first hat-trick since Sir Alex Ferguson retired in May 2013.

## 25th June 2020

The temperature continues to rise and we are enjoying a glorious summer. We dread to think how much tougher lockdown would have been if the weather had not been kind to us. Things were not as hot in nursery as you managed to avoid close, physical contact with your female peers!

Grandma and Grandad's sixtieth birthday celebrations continued. Spending time outdoors with family would not have been possible without the sunny days we were experiencing.

When you needed a wee, you took yourself off to the outside grid and dropped your pants. It is a commendable evolution you have undertaken since the end of March, something that may not have been achieved so quickly were it not for being in lockdown.

## 26th June 2020

Grandma took you to her hairdressing salon so that she could do Auntie Emma's hair. During a pandemic, hairstyles are one of the first things you stop worrying about. People are cutting and colouring their own hair and a downturn in individuals' social presentation is generally accepted across society! You have consciously bought into this carefree attitude and did not let Grandma near your mop of curls with her scissors!

The rabbits are now going out every day in the garden. You have taken a particular shine to Marble and love having her sat on your knee.

## 28th June 2020

The Wimbledon Tennis Championships should have

started today. The Covid-19 pandemic means that it is not being held for the first time in over seventy years. Another example of how history and tradition succumbs almost immediately to a contagious virus.

Leicester became the first place in the United Kingdom forced to reinstate lockdown restrictions due to the unusually high infection rates in the city. This means that residents there are, once again, only allowed to leave their homes for essential reasons.

Critics in the media are claiming that the Government relaxed the nationwide restrictions too early. It is a tough, unpredictable balance. With no recent example of a pandemic to go off, the Government has to make decisions based on the data they are presented by scientists. They also have to consider the emotional welfare of the country, which has been affected so much by lockdown.

### 1st July 2020 – One Hundredth Day in Lockdown

We cannot believe that we are in July already. Whilst this year has certainly been the strangest for all members of our household, the monotony of lockdown has not slowed time down.

We are pretty sure that you and Darcie behave all day for Grandma and Grandad and then turn feral when your parents arrive for tea. Tonight, you both thought it was wise and fair to simultaneously throw your fish pie over the lawn.

This morning, Mummy thought that it was cute that you kept asking, *Which way now, Mummy?* driving to Grandma and Grandad's. On the other hand, I found it annoyingly repetitive on the way home when you asked the same question three times in thirty seconds on a straight stretch of road. To your credit, you are starting to learn left from right!

### 3rd July 2020

I took you to Grandma's so that she could cut my hair for the first time since March. You accepted the Jelly Baby bribe so Grandma trimmed the sides of your head.

Later in the day, you followed me home in Mummy's car after picking some dining room chairs up from her friend's house. Back at our house, you claimed to be a policeman and told me off for driving too fast!

Your perception of what is potentially harmful to animals was exposed when you jumped over Marble and Quartz in the kitchen. Mummy's verbal apprehension did little to rectify your behaviour as you then proceeded to do a single step-over around Quartz's body. You were quickly removed from the situation and put in the bath!

Nana Roz and James decided to postpone their wedding, which was scheduled for 5th September. Covid-19 restrictions mean that there is a strict limit on how many people can attend such functions and they want to be able to enjoy their wedding with everyone there, whenever that may be.

*Chapter 6*

# EASING LOCKDOWN (PHASE THREE)

**4th July 2020**
Independence Day in the United States of America was dubbed 'Super Saturday' here. Pubs and restaurants were allowed to open, along with other non-essential businesses. Grandma opened her hairdressing salon to customers for the first time since March.

The Pinkfong album in Daddy's car gets some serious air time. After Track 5 – 'The Lion' – finished you shouted, *That's a good song!* In your two-year-old opinion, maybe.

We took the opportunity presented by the easing of lockdown restrictions to go to the pub for a few drinks with Kieran, Jayne and Erin. The bar was shut and drinks could only be served to tables. There was a caginess to the atmosphere and it felt so much different to what we have taken for granted as 'normal'. It was nice to drink a draught pint after all the cans and bottles we had been through since the start of spring.

### 5th July 2020

For some people, the relaxation of lockdown rules has been welcomed and they are enjoying a semblance of normality. We travelled to a pub in Addingham, near Skipton, for lunch. All bar and restaurant staff had to wear face coverings. This perplexed you and you asked, *Why are they wearing masks, there?*

Back home, you broke off from playing with your trucks in the kitchen to tell us, *It is squashed!* Whilst all God's creatures are equally precious there was an element of relief when I found out that 'it' was only a woodlouse!

### 6th July 2020

It is fascinating to see you develop so many subtle quirks. Before bed, you insist that the landing light is left on and your door is left ajar. Awakening for the day you demanded the same criteria as you thought it was still night-time. Despite constant reassurance that you had been asleep for the best part of twelve hours, it led to a very grumpy start to the day.

At nursery, you were apparently practising your *karate kicks* on the other children. We are not sure who you have picked that up from because neither of your parents are martial artists!

Wales relaxed their lockdown restrictions which have meant that, since the end of March, people have not been allowed to travel more than five miles from their home. This is a welcome relief because we have booked to go to

Wales at the end of the month. We have optimistically reserved a cottage near Caernarfon after a wedding Mummy and I were meant to be going to in Donegal, Ireland, was postponed. Disappointment awaits as when I told you where we are going you responded, *I'm going seeing some whales.*

Mummy took the rabbits to the vets and they think that Marble may actually be a boy!

**8th July 2020**
In golf, the forty-third Ryder Cup matches, scheduled to be played at Whistling Straights in Wisconsin, United States of America, at the end of September, have been postponed until 2021 due to Covid-19. Events continue to fall by the wayside. Whilst sporting events pale into insignificance during a pandemic, their cancellation dashes some hope of a return to normality.

**9th July 2020**
Two toileting accidents at nursery, along with an outfit change after 'messy play', meant that you came home in a pair of undersized, pink, frilly leggings. This look was made all the more fascinating by the fact that you paired them with your wellies!

**10th July 2020**
Today was the first time Nana Roz had looked after you on a Friday for 112 days. To place this into context the last time, on 20th March, you were 836 days old.

The rates of people in hospital testing positive for Covid-19 has fallen dramatically from 21,516 on 12th

April to 2,224 today. We were satisfied that the risk had lowered enough for normal service to resume on a Friday. For now.

You did not stop talking all day because you were so excited to be spending time with Nana Roz. You liked seeing Milly, her cat. Thankfully, you failed to notice that Pudsey is no longer with us.

### 12th July 2020

We spent the afternoon in the Ribble Valley, Lancashire, with Grandma, Grandad, Liam, Emma and Darcie.

At the castle you were preoccupied with where the dragon I told you lived there was. You insisted that I took a photo of you in the alcove of a stone window, referring to the ledge as the *dragon's bed.*

We walked down to the mill for something to drink and you steered Darcie in her pram. You needed some guidance as you struggled to touch the push bar with your outstretched arms.

I took you off for a walk and you were particularly drawn to two statues of dogs. Back at the table you unashamedly told everyone that you had *touched its willy!*

We had something to eat in a beer garden where you had been with Mummy and I when you were six months old. Back then, you sat on my knee as we went down the slide. Today, you were trying to climb up the same slide as children wanted to come down the other way!

### 14th July 2020

From 24th July, the Government will make it mandatory to wear face masks in shops. The measure is already in place on all public transport. Whilst we feel as though we are moving towards the 'New Normal', there is always the risk of a second 'spike' in Covid-19 infections.

After two not-so-good days in nursery, 'listening with your ears' is high on mine and your Mummy's agenda. Your strong mind continues to influence your behaviour as you struggle to cope with not being able to have your own way all the time!

### 15th July 2020

Great-Nana Mave's eighty-third birthday. We are so lucky that she has not caught Covid-19 as the risk to her is raised. Subconsciously, you must have known that it was her birthday as the first thing you asked for on waking up was cake!

You eventually had some cake mid-morning in the café as you and Darcie belatedly celebrated Grandma's birthday with the friends she goes walking with.

You and Darcie think that it is hilarious to *hide* from your parents as we arrive at Grandma and Grandad's for tea. Both of you have not cottoned on to the fact that we like you to hide so we can enjoy a bit of peace and quiet!

### 20th July 2020

The start of the school summer holidays. I was off work today as I should have been recovering from my friend's stag do in Munich, Germany. Being able to save money is one of the few perks of lockdown.

We went to Chatsworth House in Bakewell, Derbyshire, for a picnic and had a walk around the grounds of the stately home. You wanted to climb in the fountain and pull all the change out! Mummy and I were able to enjoy a stop at a pub on the way home as you slept all the way.

We will be spending a lot of time in my car over the next few weeks as we have got trips to Wales and Cornwall planned. However, infection rates are rising across the country. The town where we live is third in the country on the list of infections per 100,000 people according to data collected between 12th and 16th July.

**21st July 2020**

Even though Mummy is off for the summer we have decided to send you into nursery every Tuesday. The reintegration after the first few months of lockdown was a tough one for you and we want to help you avoid the same feelings of anxiety come September.

As Mummy and I had our tea, we left you watching television in the front room. All was well until you walked into the kitchen, felt-tip pen in hand, declaring, *Noah drawed on the couches!* Suppose that will teach me not to leave my case of Sharpie pens lying around!

I shaved my beard for the first time since lockdown began. At the start of the pandemic, I pledged not to get rid of it until we were out the other side. My scraggy face had almost become a symbol of the times we were living through. With no end in sight, it was time to smarten up! One small consolation was that it pleased Mummy.

**24th July 2020**

An unexpected start to the day as I woke up, in the early hours, with pains radiating from my chest and down my arms. Mummy had to drive me to the hospital which meant you had to come too. You were oblivious to the fact that I may have been having a heart attack, suffering a blood clot or both!

Having been to bed, and awakened, in daylight hours for more than three months, the darkness fascinated you. *I can see lots of streetlights… I can see one star… Look! Lights flashing in the trees!*

You and Mummy could not come into the hospital which meant I had to go and sit alone. The hospital waiting room had an eerie feeling to it. The nurses paced about in masks, gloves and aprons and the patients sat spaced apart around the waiting room. There were screens erected everywhere to try and prevent the transmission of the virus.

I got home shortly after 5am, discharged with no concerns. You thought that the red ECG pads on my hairy chest were stickers and tried to pull them off!

**25th July 2020**
We looked after Darcie for the day so Liam and Emma could enjoy some time together. Driving to Blackburn to see one of Mummy's friends, Darcie taught you the words and actions to 'Let It Go' from the Disney film *Frozen*. The amateur dramatics from the pair of you waving your arms around in your car seats were very amusing!

Those that do not know you think you are twins, with your curly blonde hair, blue eyes and extremely close bond.

Back at home, Kieran and Jayne called round with baby Erin and you showed her your bunny rabbits. You attempted to pick Marble up and he jumped down from the top level of the garden, landing awkwardly. This led to some 'time out', but luckily Marble was fine.

### 26th July 2020

Auntie Stevie's twenty-seventh birthday.

Early in the afternoon we went to see the Finnys. My 'cousin' Holly, lives in Dubai and had been unable to travel back to the country until now because of Covid-19 travel restrictions.

My other 'cousin' Dani's son Joseph is four and starts school in September. It was a great test for you playing football with him as you are used to being the one who makes up all the rules!

We went to Auntie Stevie and Uncle Simon's for tea. Harley has become accustomed to you and your little character. Your face was a picture when she jumped up and licked your face. *No, Harley!* you whined, wiping your cheeks with your hand.

It was the final day of the Premier League season. United beat Leicester 2–0 and finished third in the league. Liverpool won their nineteenth English league title some time ago and finished the season seventeen points clear of Manchester City on ninety-nine points.

The Government performed a U-turn regarding travel to Spain. Due to a spike in Covid-19 cases in the country, all Brits there currently will have to self-isolate for two weeks when they return home. A sign of how quickly things can change during a pandemic.

### 27th July 2020

As I opened the back door to put out the recycling I spotted Marble lying in an abnormal position at the bottom of his hutch. Trying to ignore my immediate feelings of dread, I went to have a look at him. Sadly, Marble was dead.

Mummy also did not want to believe that he had passed away. She kept you busy as I put him in a box to take him to the vet's on my way to work.

The vet later confirmed that Marble had suffered trauma to his back, probably caused by when he jumped to escape you on Saturday. Marble was cremated and his ashes were scattered at a place in the hills where the vet takes animals after they have died.

It was devastatingly sad, and so difficult, to explain to you what had happened to Marble. I told you that Marble had been poorly and taken to live in the hills with the other poorly 'bunny rabbits'.

Mummy and I choked back tears as you repeatedly asked, *Why?* You could not comprehend why Marble no longer lived in his hutch with Quartz. *Where's Quartz's friend? Why?*

You played with Quartz in the kitchen, cuddling him and resting your head on his back. Your display of bewilderment and innocence was so upsetting as you were not to know, or understand, how your actions had most certainly caused Marble harm.

Marble's passing obviously paled into insignificance when considering the wider devastation so many people around the world have, and still are, experiencing due to the Covid-19 pandemic. Admittedly, Marble's death was a trivial microcosm, but the saddest day of lockdown for us so far. Especially considering how much you loved him in the short time he was with us.

Chapter 7

# THE LLŶN PENINSULA, NORTH WALES

**30th July 2020**

Today, Mummy and I should have been leaving you at home with grandparents whilst we went to Donegal, Ireland, for a wedding. As it was cancelled due to Covid-19, we took the opportunity to go and stay in one of Mummy's friend's cottages in North Wales.

*We're off! We're off! We're off in a motor car!* you sang on the way to our first stop at Cheshire Oaks Designer Outlet. You wanted to stretch your legs a bit too far when we got there and kept running off from me, in and out of the shops. *Don't shout at me!* you ordered after I decided to pick you up to keep you safe.

We then went to the Blue Planet Aquarium, which you loved! You knew all the different sea creatures from the books and television programmes you have immersed yourself in. Your favourite, unsurprisingly, were the sharks and you remarked that they had *toothy grins*, a reference to the Julia Donaldson book, *The Snail and the Whale*.

It was a year to the day since we flew to Greece on our last family holiday. You are too young to remember that but we wondered if, on this holiday, you might make some of your earliest memories.

As we pulled up outside our holiday cottage you moaned, pointing at the sea, *Don't want to go on holiday! Want to see some whales over there!* You have still not quite worked out that Wales is a country.

As Mummy and I enjoyed some peace, watching a film, we heard a loud thud upstairs. You had fallen through the two single beds we had pushed together for you! Thankfully, the only impact it had was to disrupt your sleep for a minute or two.

Before we went to bed, news filtered through that lockdown restrictions had been tightened in our area. We are no longer allowed family and friends in our homes.

## 31st July 2020

We have been given lots of recommendations for the three days we are here so we were up early and off to the beach in Llanbedrog.

The temperature of the sea put you off going in initially but you were soon playing your own game of fetch, throwing a rock into the water and chasing after it.

The Covid-19 restrictions have not been relaxed in Wales to the same extent they have in England. The queue snaked around the side of the beach café so we drove to Abersoch for lunch. You chose turkey dinosaurs and spent more time playing with them than you did eating. A t-rex, stegosaurus and triceratops did not satisfy you enough so you asked the waitress, *Where's the pterodactyl?*

We had promised you that we would go crabbing so it was back in the car for a drive to Porthmadog. Mummy and I took it in turns casting the lines over the harbour wall to prevent you from toppling in! We caught lots of crabs, or *crabbings* as you called them! You helped to scoop them into the bucket with your net as we lifted them out of the water.

'Who's the best at crabbing, Noah? Me or Mummy', I enquired.

*Me!* you confidently responded.

Back at the cottage I played football with you in the garden. You were willing to head the ball for the first time.

Before bed, we played board games with you. This was funny as you had no concept of waiting for your turn! Mummy tried to drum this into you by making you put your hands on your knees!

### 1st August 2020

*What's the princess doing in there?* you asked, pointing at the church across the road from the cottage. You are convinced that the church is a castle and, to be fair, it is a fine example of architecture.

First stop today was Nefyn and District Golf Club which we walked across to Porthdinllaen Beach. A wayward drive, followed by a shout of 'Fore!', upset you somewhat. *Don't like fore!*

We followed the coastal path to the lifeboat station where we saw what we set out to see – seals! You were really good at spotting them bobbing up and down in the waves.

At Gypsy Wood Park you were adamant that you did not want to go on the train ride so it was a relief that we had two hours to convince you otherwise! We had a look at the animals and a donkey ride was another thing that you did not fancy! Walking through the wetlands in your new, flashing wellies you kept telling me *It's only mud, Dad!* as you happily jumped through the puddles.

Driving back you dozed off so I pulled into a pub car park off a busy roundabout. Mummy watched you from the seating area outside as I bought us a drink each to enjoy, quietly, in the sun.

When we got back the FA Cup Final was on television. You kept asking me *Where's Bruno?* I had to explain that Bruno Fernandes was not playing because Chelsea had knocked United out in the semi-finals. Arsenal won 2–1, to lift a record-extending FA Cup.

We tried board games again at bedtime and you played snakes and ladders with Mummy. Contrary to the aim of the game, you got more excited when landing on a snake than you did a ladder!

### 2$^{nd}$ August 2020

I had been 'threatening' to feed you to the Welsh dragon for bouts of misbehaviour. This meant you were petrified when we got to Caernarfon Castle as this is where you thought the dragon lived!

You chose to buy a Welsh rugby ball in the souvenir shop and spent the next half an hour walking around the town centre with it clutched under your arm.

We crossed the Britannia Bridge into Anglesey for the afternoon, where I had enjoyed holidays with Grandma and Grandad as a child. In Rhosneigr, where we ate fish and chips for lunch, you were insistent that the sea was a *river*.

Moving on to Trearddur Bay, where your Great-Grandma Buckley used to spend her summers, we realised how much more difficult it was to get a drink in Wales. We were not able to get in the hotel or restaurants without a reservation.

On the way back we stopped off in Beaumaris to partake in a spot of your new-found, favourite pastime – crabbing! You walked the streets, holding your pink fishing net, telling anyone who would listen where you were going.

Walking across the pebbled beach to crab under Beaumaris pier, we told you that a dead crab was 'asleep'. As you trudged to your next crabbing adventure you announced you wanted to *catch a morning crab*. Presumably, this was your way of saying you wanted to catch a crab that was awake!

Standing on the beams under the pier was a lot more successful than we thought it was going to be and we caught a bucketful of crabs. You and Mummy won the competition of who could catch the biggest!

### 3rd **August 2020**
*Bye-bye, house! Bye-bye, castle! Bye-bye, Princess! Bye-bye, shop! Bye-bye, mountain!* Evidently, you had become quite attached to your surroundings during our four-night stay in North Wales!

We broke the journey home up with a stop at Knowsley Safari Park. Once there, you transferred to Mummy's knee in the front of the car for a better vantage point of the animals. I took a chance and chose to drive the riskier route through the baboon enclosure. That cost me my back windscreen wiper as a group of baboons ripped it off. You and Mummy were much more amused than I was. *Look, Daddy! Monkey's eating it! Me go get it!* Thanks for the offer, Little Man, but you are staying where you are!

On the foot safari we saw some *merry cats* (meercats), a tiger and – Mummy's favourite – some giraffes! As we watched vultures, owls and kites at the 'Birds of Prey' show, swooping down to eat meaty treats, you became distracted by a far-less interesting avian, excitedly shouting, *Look! A seagull!*

As we pulled up on the drive at home you woke up and cried, *Don't want to go in my house! Want to go back to Wales!*

### 4th **August 2020**

On the way home from nursery, Mummy took you to the shop to buy Quartz some greens. You carried the spinach to the till and informed the lady serving you, *It's for Quartz... not Marble. Marble poorly... gone to the hills.* Then, after a brief pause, *I threw it!* Whilst your interpretation of the events which caused Marble's injury, and subsequent death, was incorrect, it hinted at a higher level of understanding then we first thought.

You took Harley for a walk in the park and two overweight pugs jumping up at Mummy caused you to ask, *What are them piggies doing?* Haha!

Chapter 8

# DEVON, CORNWALL AND THE MIDLANDS

**7th August 2020**
Mummy dragged you out of bed at 4.55am, much to your anguish. The plan was for you to fall back asleep on the journey to Weston-Super-Mare for breakfast. That did not happen as you chatted to us the whole way there.

We arrived in Plymouth at around midday and went for a walk through Hoe Park and down to the Barbican. *What's the lighthouse doing there?* you enquired.

Eating lunch at the harbour, I tried to trick you into eating some crab by putting it on the end of your fish finger. Fooled you were not, picking it off and throwing it back on my plate!

Your good behaviour in the restaurant earnt you an ice cream. You chose a mixed-berry sorbet but asked the young lady at the counter for a *mixed sorry babe!*

We went to a Greek restaurant in the evening. The

couple on the table next to us were mesmerised by your cheeky character. You were rolling the foil wrappers off your chocolates and throwing them on the floor for the man to pick up for you!

**8$^{th}$ August 2020**
The Penthouse, where breakfast was served in the hotel, had fantastic views across Hoe Park and The Sound. The service, on the other hand, was not so delightful. Due to Covid-19, we had to queue for the hot buffet. Waiting twenty-five minutes to get food is not so fun when you have a hungry two-year-old in tow!

After we checked out you wanted to play minigolf. So eager were you to get started you helped the woman put the last few flags out on the course. Your putting technique was more akin to sliding a hockey puck along. I found the pace of the greens a bit too slow but Mummy got a hole-in-one!

We met Grandma, Grandad, Liam, Emma and Darcie in Trebarwith Strand, Cornwall, for lunch. Afterwards, we spent a short time on the beach where Grandma Buckley used to play as a child. Then, we travelled to a house in Newquay which we had rented for the week.

Before lockdown, you had been going for swimming lessons every Saturday morning. You were confident and loved being in the water. Having missed swimming for almost five months, you did not want to get in the pool in the back garden.

**10$^{th}$ August 2020**
No one needs to set a morning alarm when Darcie is up

at 7am! This is something we are not used to as you love a lie-in!

We were packed up and ready for a day at Crantock beach at 9.30am. As the tide drew back out down the estuary it left shallow pools in the quicksand which you and Darcie loved splashing in.

Grandad then took you to the top of a steep sand dune and, for some unknown reason, thought it was a good idea to let go of your hand so you could run down! After half a dozen steps you lost your footing and rolled the next few yards down the hill. When you picked yourself up your face, nostrils, mouth and ears were full of sand. Despite claiming you were dizzy, you said that you enjoyed it! The whole escapade caused Grandad to be very sheepish for the next few hours!

We spent the rest of the afternoon by the pool at the house. It is now two days running that we have tried to coax you into the water, only to be met with kicking and screaming. Darcie is doing really well, swimming on her own. Whilst this is largely inconsequential, it is an example of how lockdown can affect an individual's social and emotional development and confidence. It is strange how a few months away from swimming has led to you becoming fearful of the water. Hopefully, you will have shaken it off before the end of the week.

United beat FC Copenhagen 1–0, after extra-time, in the quarter-finals of the UEFA Europa League. The last three stages of the tournament are being played behind closed doors in Germany. The quarter- and semi-finals are taking place over one leg, instead of the usual two, due to Covid-19.

### 12th August 2020

The weather has been overcast for most of the week. We decided to chase the sun and drive to the beach at Bude. Many people had the same idea and the beach was very busy.

We managed to bag a table in the beach bar for lunch. Table service and ordering food and drink through mobile-phone apps is taking some getting used to. It certainly does not lend itself to a relaxing experience. You sat on a stool next to Grandad and were drawn to videos of people surfing on the television – *What's them waves doing there? What's them people doing?*

Having been in the pool at the house yesterday, you were happy jumping the waves with Darcie and Grandad. You both referred to the waves as *speed bumps*!

### 13th August 2020

You and Darcie got your wish of travelling to Land's End together in Grandad's car. We passed you on the journey as you had pulled into a lay-by so you could empty your bladder onto Grandad's back tyre!

When we all arrived you were running around excitedly and jumped into a puddle, splashing an unsuspecting tourist! Luckily, they also saw the funny side!

On the cliffs near the famous signpost at Land's End you took a great photograph of me and Mummy. Usually, they are blurred with body parts cut out of the frame but this one had us both in the middle of the shot!

We stopped off at one of my favourite beaches in the world at Porthcurno on the way back. A one-way system had been installed on the hill for people to use on the way to and from the beach. The backlog you caused through insisting you help me pull the beach trolley created some embarrassment as people patiently waited behind us.

Back at the house you took an interest in watching a sport new to you – snooker. You constantly asked questions as the players potted different coloured balls, one after another. Snooker is one of the first sports that has reintroduced spectators during the pandemic.

### 14th August 2020

The crabbing in Cornwall has definitely not been as fruitful as it was in Anglesey, with unsuccessful attempts in Bude, Newquay and, this morning, Padstow.

You have now started to make links between the strange goings-on in the world and the Covid-19 virus. With the country, and wider world, consumed by the virus and the news associated with it, you have started to process information yourself. Walking away from an inflatable park, you pointed at a motorbike and said, *Virus running Mummy over*. Perhaps you have overheard how the virus is killing people? Pressed on this, you assured us that you are not scared of the virus.

As it was our last night, we all ate out at an Australian restaurant. Once we had eaten, you and Darcie had your first taste of 'gambling', at an amusement arcade, on the 2p machines. You both won a tub of bubbles and soon found out that you cannot use the soapy lotion once it has been emptied onto the floor!

### 15th August 2020

As you were leaving our *holiday house*, as you have referred to for the last week, Darcie asked where you were going.

You told her, *We are going to Frankie's house*, and she said that she wanted to come with you!

It took almost six hours to drive from Cornwall to the Midlands, where our friends, Chris, Romy and their one-year-old boy, Frankie, live.

We walked out to eat in a beer garden soon after we arrived. You and Frankie ate pizza for tea, but not after an almighty row. Who knew how much upset could be caused by wanting to play with the same Morrison's HGV toy!

You have learnt to pretend that you are sulking, with your trademark mock frown and protruding bottom lip. This is usually countered by either me or Mummy tapping your lip with our finger, which causes you to break into a smile. There was no way this method was going to remedy this particular tantrum as tears and snot flew everywhere!

**16th August 2020**

After spending the day with Chris, Romy and Frankie – going to the park, playing minigolf and having some lunch – we drove the last leg of the 952 miles we have covered home.

You were so excited to see Quartz! Again, you asked about Marble and, in a conversation with Mummy, you told her that he had jumped and hurt himself. I do not think we will ever find out the full details of what happened to him.

United's prolonged season ended 371 days after it started, with a 2–1 semi-final defeat in the Europa League to Sevilla. When we watched the first game of the 2019/20 season in Greece, a 4–0 home win against Chelsea on 11th August 2019, we could never have imagined what would unfold over the months that have followed.

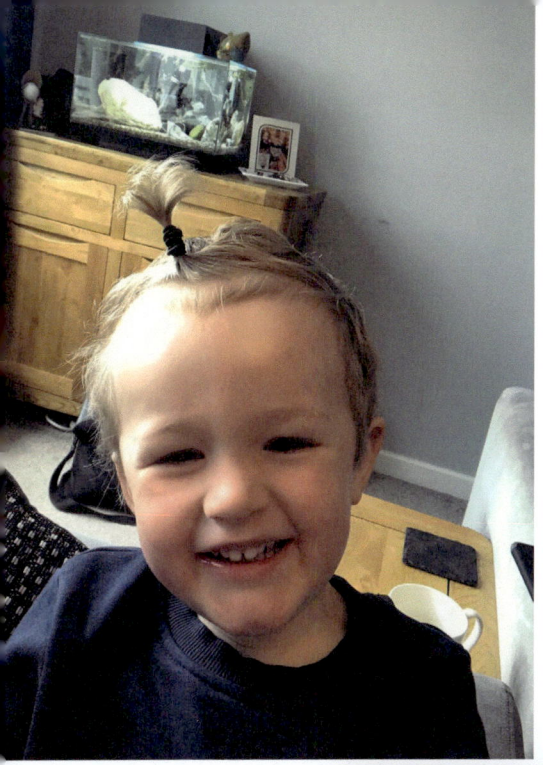

*This is what happened the first time I left you alone with Mummy to go in work after we were told to 'stay at home'.*

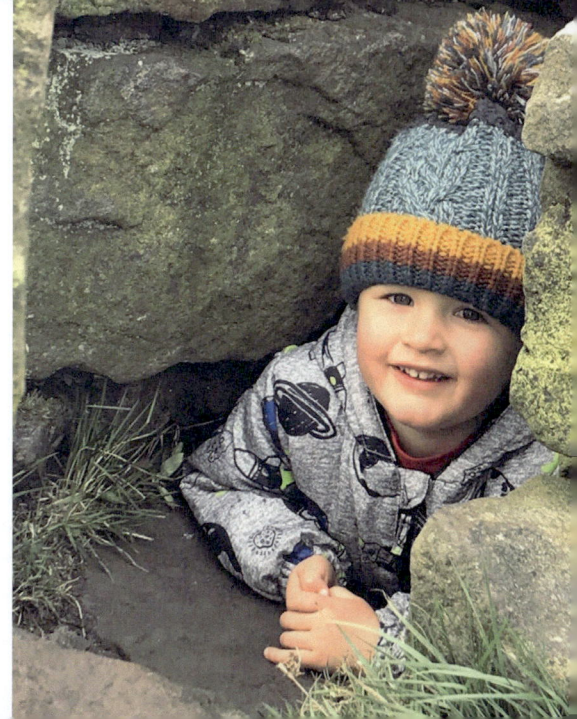

*Posing at the gate near the alpacas. We were so lucky to have such great countryside around where we lived where we could enjoy our daily walks.*

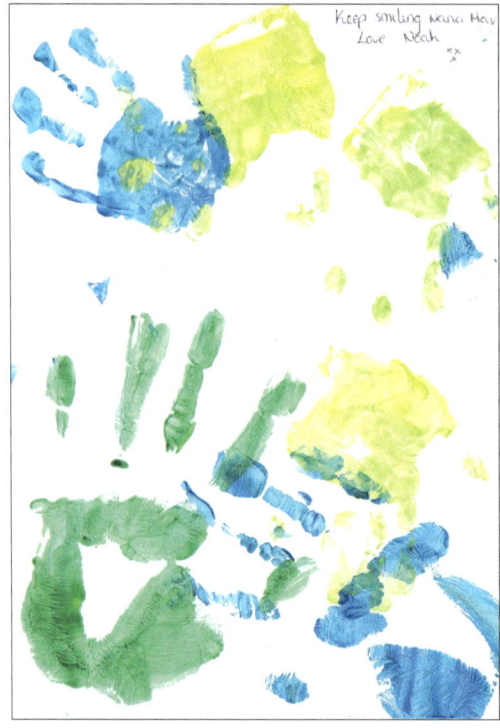

*Some hand art you did for Great Nana Mave. It was difficult to adjust to not seeing family members at the start of lockdown.*

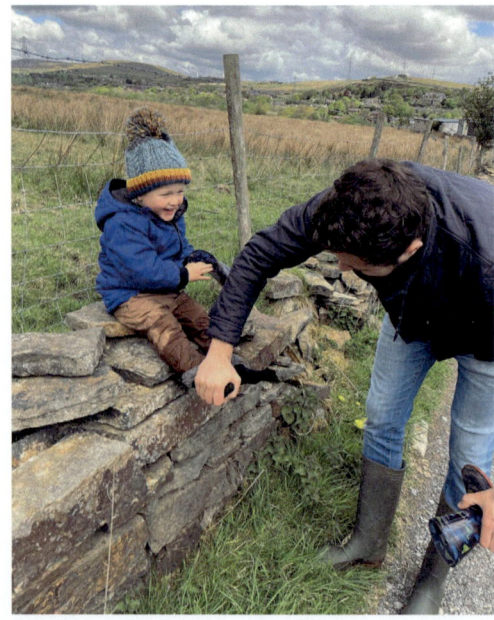

*Giggling as I wring water out of your sock. You were a typical toddler full of adventure and mischief!*

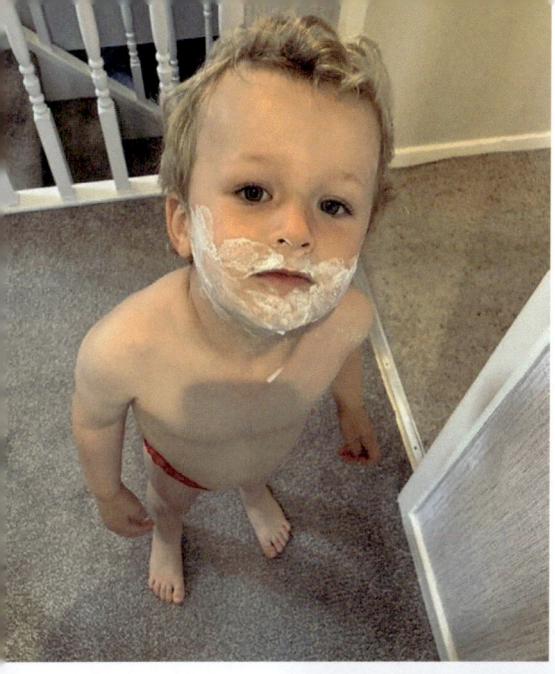

*Curious after I shaved my neck, you wanted to give it a try. Walking round the house in your underwear was a common sight in lockdown.*

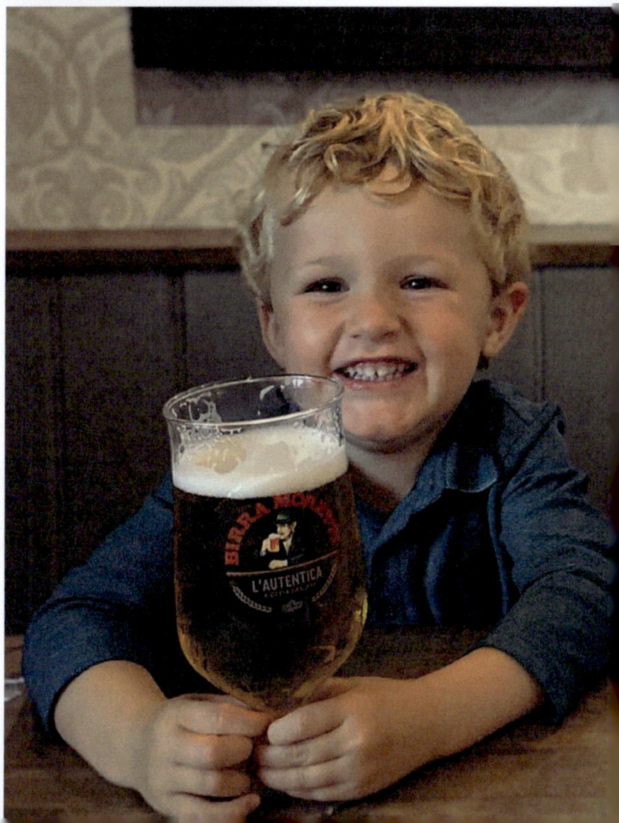

*'Super Saturday' in the pub. Table service and having to remain seated in bars and restaurants became a part of the 'new normal'.*

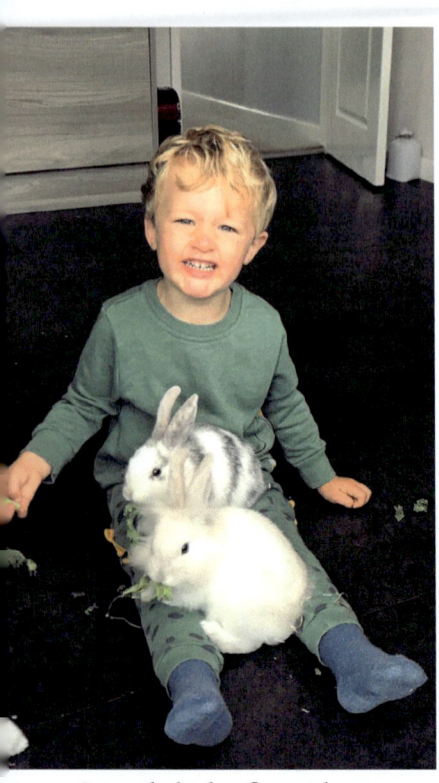

*Sat on the kitchen floor with your new bunnies – Marble and Quartz. Tragically, Marble was not with us for long.*

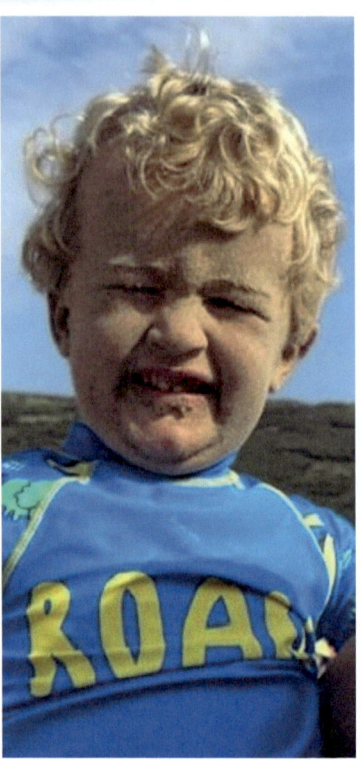

*Your face after Grandad Col walked you to the top of a steep sand dune and let you make your own way down!*

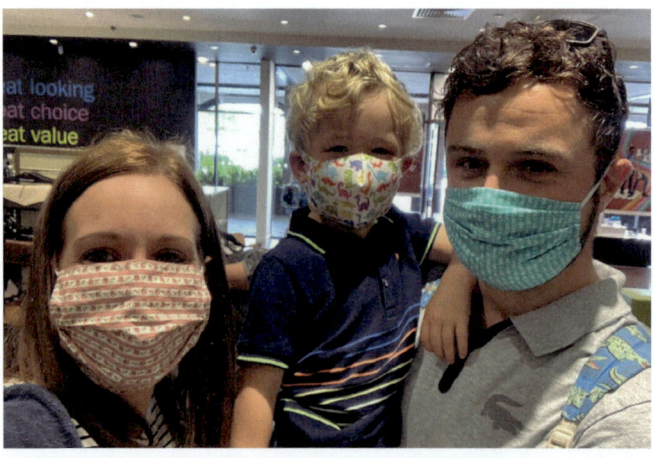

*At the end of July 2020, it became essential to wear face coverings in shops.*

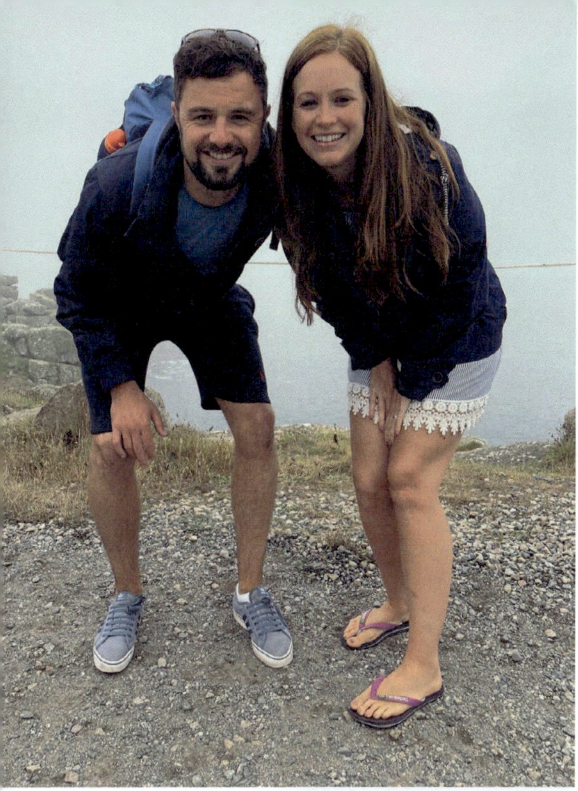

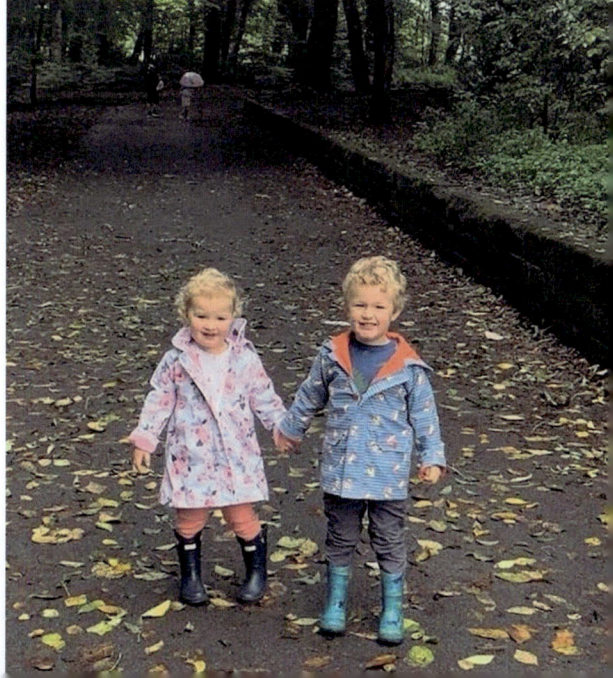

*You took this picture of Mummy and I at Land's End. Admittedly, there were a few outtakes prior.*

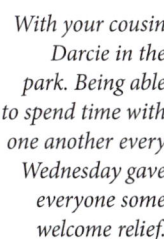

*With your cousin Darcie in the park. Being able to spend time with one another every Wednesday gave everyone some welcome relief.*

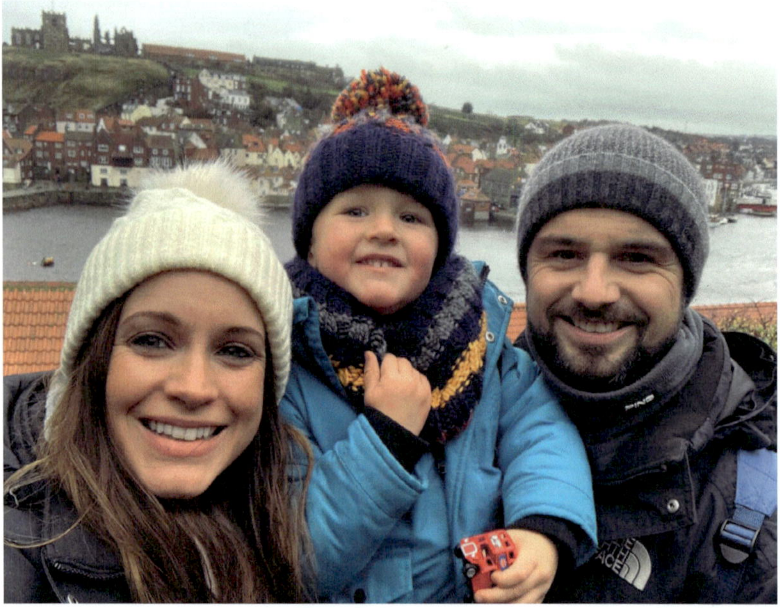

*A family selfie in Whitby before the long, dark winter of 2020. The 'Vampire's Castle' is in the top left.*

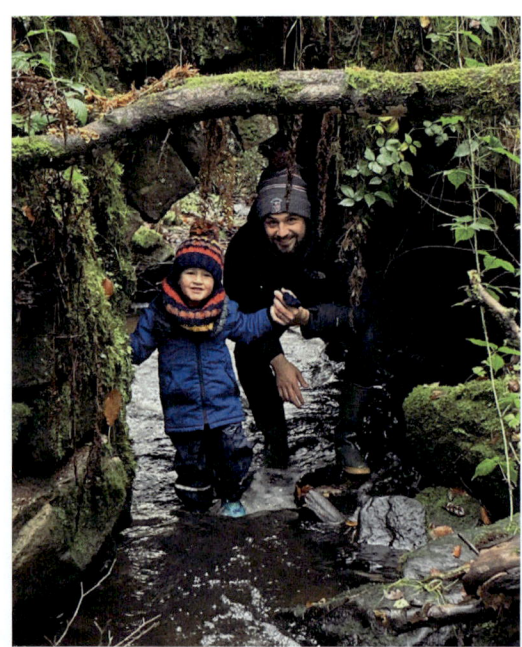

*In the 'Gruffalo's Cave'. You loved relating your story books to things we came across on our walks. Disappointingly for you, there were no hippos in that stream!*

Chapter 9

# LOCAL LOCKDOWN CONTINUES

**19th August 2020**
Soaking up information and learning new things is all part and parcel of being a toddler. After tea, your curiosity extended to your own anatomy.

Having done a wee on your potty you stood up, willy in hand, and asked me and Mummy, *Why's my willy hard?* I walked off, leaving your Mummy to answer!

**20th August 2020 – 150 Days Since Lockdown Began**
Mummy took you for a day out with her friend Lucy and your friends Eric and Arthur. All the way there you talked about the makes and models of the vehicles on the road and counted the bridges.

After work, I took you to the golf club. You walked into the professionals' shop, palms upturned, arms stretched out in front of you and made your position clear, *I have got no golf club!* I asked one of the professionals to cut down and re-grip an old club, which you were chuffed with. We went to test it out on the grass but you soon wanted to use my pitching wedge as you claimed your club was too heavy. You were even more disappointed that the practice range did not have any holes cut out in the grass for you!

### 21st August 2020

I was up early to go and play golf in Scotland for four days. You wanted to join me and stood asking questions at the front door for twenty minutes as I got my stuff together.

I played at four different courses on the trip, including Prestwick, the venue of the first Open Championship, and the Ailsa at Turnberry, the venue for four Open Championships and owned by the current President of the United States, Donald Trump.

You were very busy with Mummy whilst I was away golfing with friends. We almost suffered the loss of another rabbit as Quartz somehow managed to escape into next door's garden.

We missed one another but spoke every day on video call. Each time, you immediately questioned where the *golf flag* was!

### 29th August 2020

The August Bank Holiday weekend at the golf club is usually reserved for the Captain's Final, a thirty-six-hole competition held over two days. This is a singles' competition and your best three scores from six qualifying rounds count towards trying to secure your entry.

Due to the pandemic, and the start of the season being wiped out, the Captain's Final was converted into a doubles' competition you did not have to qualify for. This was imaginatively named 'Not the Captain's Final'. Perhaps, less sensitively, the trophy for winning was an oversized golf ball with spikes sticking out of it – a depiction of the Covid-19 virus under a microscope.

### 31$^{st}$ August 2020 – One Thousand Days Since You Were Born

August Bank Holiday Monday, the last bank holiday until Christmas Day. We wondered what the pandemic, with its ever-changing lockdown restrictions, daily news bulletins and fluctuating infection rates will have in store for us between now and then?

We went for a walk near our house for the first time in a while. Some of the footpaths had overgrown throughout the summer months and others were fenced off completely. You cried out for help as your wellies got stuck in the mud and Mummy had to pull you out.

Later in the day, we went to the park after adjusting the seat on your balance bike. You were not too sure to begin with, tentatively trying to ride your bike whilst complaining it was *too wobbly*!

Chapter 10

# THE 'NEW NORMAL'?

**1st September 2020**
Mummy returned to work in the classroom for the first time in 165 days. Due to the Covid-19 pandemic, the school day looks a lot different to how it was at the beginning of March. The children have staggered start times, parents and visitors are not allowed into school and different year groups, referred to as 'bubbles', are not allowed to mix with one another.

Mummy works in a different town to where we live and there are stricter lockdown restrictions there. This means that Mummy has to wear a visor, covering her face, everywhere except the classroom.

The threat of a 'second wave' of Covid-19, as we move into winter, looms large. The measures imposed in schools are designed to keep the R rate down. In a few weeks, schools may be forced to close again if the transmission of the virus increases.

**2nd September 2020**

Comedy moment of the day? Refusing to listen to advice when climbing on the back of Grandma and Grandad's dining room chair before it fell on top of you! The shock and light crush set you off into floods of tears. Luckily, when we asked where it hurt you only pointed to the tip of your nose!

**3rd September 2020**

Comedy moment of the day? After going for a wee on your own at nursery, one of the staff heard you shouting her name repeatedly from inside the cubicle. She opened the door to find you folded up inside the toilet basin!

Low moment of the day? Emptying your bladder all over the sofa as you watched television before bed. Due to your nonchalance and cheek that followed, if I would have had my way, you would not have had the bedtime story Mummy read to you. You cried, *I want to be a good boy!* as Mummy informed you that your punishment was not getting a bedtime song.

At times, it is heart-breaking being a toddler but just as heart-wrenching trying to parent one!

**5th September 2020**

Today should have been Nana Roz and James' wedding day. Another casualty of Covid-19. It has been postponed until next year when things should hopefully be back to normal.

**6th September 2020**

We visited our friends Planty, Vicky and baby Grace, who had recently celebrated her first birthday. The odd time, we have asked you if you would like a baby sibling. Your consistent answer is, *No… a Gruffalo!*

In the afternoon, we went for Sunday lunch with the rest of the Buckley family. You and Darcie were very well behaved, occupied with colouring pictures and playing with toys. Privacy and dignity is still something you are working on. Walking across the restaurant, you announced to an elderly lady, *I'm going for a poo!*

The Government reported 2,988 new cases of Covid-19 today. This is the highest number of daily cases since May. Is this an early indication that the second wave of Covid-19 is imminent?

**9th September 2020**

Since Cornwall, you have often told us how you would like to go back to our *holiday house*. We are hoping to book a week in Turkey at the end of October but that all depends on the Covid-19 travel restrictions closer to the time.

There is now a list that the Government has drawn up which stipulates which countries you can travel to without having to self-isolate for fourteen days on returning to the United Kingdom. Countries are added to, and removed from, the list on an almost weekly basis.

The Government announced that from Monday 14th September it will be illegal for groups of more than six to gather anywhere, indoors or outdoors, until further notice. The lack of a predicted timeframe for the duration of this new measure is most definitely worrying.

**11th September 2020**

Last night, you had a sleepover at Nana Roz and James'

house. A 5.30am wake-up call was not what James ordered on the morning of his sixtieth birthday. You stood on the landing making a fuss about the fact that the bed you had woken up in was not yours.

When you came home, you were suffering from a cold. You have suffered a few injuries during lockdown, as a result of being a boisterous little boy, but this was the first time you have had as much as a sniffle.

### 12th September 2020

I brought a horse chestnut – 'conker' – back from my morning run for you. You clearly did not remember what they were from last year, when you rolled the smooth brown nuts around the floor in the kitchen.

Mummy and I went to a wedding in the Forest of Bowland. Despite Covid-19, the wedding was allowed to go ahead with a maximum of thirty guests permitted at the ceremony. Confetti was not permitted and dancing was banned. The room was partitioned off during the wedding reception to make it look like two separate parties. We are not too sure what would have happened if it was not, as the police turned up at the rural venue during the meal to check the regulations were being adhered to.

### 13th September 2020

Your enthusiasm for 'conkers' is now back so we went to the park to knock some out of the trees. It was too early in the autumn as they were still white when we opened their green, prickly cases.

After tea, you did yet another wee on the sofa. When asked why, your candid response was, *'Cos* (of) *the virus!*

For all the medical information we have consumed about Covid-19, we are pretty sure that the virus does not cause you to wet yourself! For the first time since May, 3,000 Covid-19 cases were recorded for the third consecutive day. It certainly feels as though the virus is starting to take a hold on daily life again. The total number of deaths from Covid-19 in the country since the start of the pandemic is 41,628.

**17<sup>th</sup> September 2020**

Your day at nursery took a turn for the worse when you pulled your friend Hazel's hair. Apparently, your justification was that you were not happy she was walking away from you. I suppose that is one way to halt someone in their tracks!

We are now required to supervise you even more closely in the garden as you have figured out how to let Quartz out of his hutch.

The north east of England went into lockdown again. For people living there, this means they cannot socialise with anyone outside of their household. There are also much tighter restrictions in pubs and restaurants. It feels inevitable that changes to the lockdown rules in our area will be imposed soon.

**19<sup>th</sup> September 2020**

Uncle Liam's thirty-second birthday.

As I left the house to go to golf you asked me, *Are you going to get it in the hole? Are you going to go 'swoosh', like that?!* whilst imitating a golf swing with your arms.

Mummy took you to a watch an outdoor show

with Lucy and Eric. You were scared of the pirates and reluctantly watched them through floods of tears! The only time you stopped gripping Mummy tightly was to get up and dance to 'Let It Go' and 'Baby Shark'.

United lost their first game of the Premier League season, 3–1 at home to Crystal Palace. New signing, Donny van de Beek, came off the bench to score a consolation goal. Fans are still not allowed in stadiums to watch games but authorities are considering trialling this from 1st October.

**20th September 2020**
Driving past the hospital, we told you that was where you were born. Gazing at the sprawling building from your car seat, you murmured, *Yeah… hospital.*

A minute later, I asked you where you had come out of Mummy's tummy. Hilariously, you answered, *In Tesco!*

The 'Rule of Six', which came into effect at the start of the week, means that people from different households are not allowed to socialise in groups of more than six. With lockdown having an unparalleled impact on the lives of everyone in the country, people do find ways of getting round them in a desperate effort to continue to live 'normally'. At the restaurant we ate in for tea, it was clear that there were groups larger than six together. They were just sat on two tables adjacent to one another.

Bending the lockdown restrictions is something that has crept into the psyche of many people up and down the country. The constraints imposed as a result of Covid-19 actually encroaches on people's human rights. It is only natural for people to want to lead as normal a life as possible, whilst trying to be respectful of the severity of the virus.

## 22nd September 2020

We are now almost six months into lockdown. At 8pm, the prime minister addressed the nation through our television screens. The number of Covid-19 infections is increasing at an alarming rate.

Boris Johnson announced that new lockdown restrictions were being imposed. This means that it is mandatory to wear face masks in shops. Pubs and restaurants must close at 10pm and wedding party sizes have been reduced to fifteen people. Plans to start allowing spectators into sporting events on 1st October have been postponed.

The prime minister maintained that the tightening of restrictions was absolutely necessary to prevent a lockdown similar to the one imposed in March. There is a suggestion that these current restraints could be in place for six months, or until a vaccination against the virus is developed.

## Chapter 11

# SUPPRESSING THE VIRUS

**26th September 2020**
Mummy's thirty-fourth birthday.

You 'bought' her a cushion with a photo of you and me on the beach in Bude printed on it. Mummy found this a lot funnier than it was intended to be!

You had been excited to go to Grandma and Grandad's all week for a sleepover. You played on their back lawn with your custom-made 7-iron from the golf club.

Mummy and I went for an afternoon out to celebrate her birthday. We had to sign into every restaurant, bar and pub as part of the 'Track and Trace' policy. First introduced in May, this was brought in so that people could be contacted if someone else in the venue later tested positive for Covid-19. All of this information is stored and shared on the NHS mobile phone app.

Face coverings had to be worn and we could only

remove them when we sat down. Food and drink had to be served to tables. The restrictions certainly impacted the atmosphere usually associated with going out. The mood was dampened and in some places it felt more like being in a hospital or a doctor's surgery.

**29<sup>th</sup> September 2020**
Today, the number of Covid-19 deaths worldwide reached one million. This is similar to the number of people who died from Asian flu in 1957 and 1958, and Hong Kong flu ten years later. Spanish flu, in 1918 and 1919, infected almost a third of the world's population and killed approximately fifty million people.

You will be catching a cold soon if you do not let us move your fan out of your bedroom. It has been in there since the summer and you are adamant it needs to be turned on every night before you go to sleep!

**30<sup>th</sup> September 2020**
Your new morning routine involves having a wash, brushing your teeth and then staring at CBeebies in a trance! You also make your own bed, put your pyjamas under your pillow and get dressed before coming downstairs.

I told you off after you wet yourself, for the third time in an hour, at Grandma and Grandad's house. Brazenly, you mimicked me back, *I'm going to get cross!*

Grandad predicted that we will be back in full lockdown come December. In the context of everything that's going on, it is a realistic proposition.

**1ˢᵗ October 2020**

Every Thursday, I pick you up from nursery. We called at the supermarket on the way home. I was entertained watching you throw the softer items over your head into the trolley without looking. This was until you snatched a jar of chilli powder out of my hand. Cue red dust and glass all over the floor!

Countries continue to move between the Green, Amber and Red lists for international travel to and from the United Kingdom. If a country is on the Red List then people have to self-isolate at home for two weeks on their return to the country. As of Saturday 3ʳᵈ October, Turkey will be added to the Red List. We feel relieved that we held off booking a holiday there at the end of the month. This means that people already there on holiday will be returning under different conditions to when they travelled abroad.

**2ⁿᵈ October 2020**

Donald Trump, the President of the United States of America, and his wife, Melania Trump, both tested positive for Covid-19. Across the 'pond', over 200,000 people have died from the virus.

I brought a few 'conkers' back from my run and left them on the front doorstep. You believed that these were delivered by a *kind squirrel*.

You had fun with me, putting a sock on each hand and making them talk to one another. You laughed so hard, you wet yourself. We let you off for that one!

**6ᵗʰ October 2020**

I had to collect you from nursery at lunchtime because

staff said that you had developed a rash on your face. On my arrival, there was not much of a rash to see. Frustratingly, we wonder whether nursery would have sent you home if they knocked the afternoon's fees off our monthly bill!

In the pharmacy, an Olaf teddy from the *Frozen* film was sat on the shelf wearing a mask. You pointed at him and asked me if he had coronavirus.

You confidently told the pharmacist, *I don't want medicine... I'm not poorly.* Your self-assessment added to my angst that I had taken a break from my busy work schedule to bring you home for the afternoon.

Darcie was sent home from nursery yesterday because she had a cough. Liam and Emma took Covid-19 tests, which both returned negative results.

### 8th October 2020

The weekly food shop with you continues to be entertaining. An elderly gentleman remarked to me, 'You don't need a shopping list with him', after hearing you shout out everything you recognised in the fruit-and-veg aisle!

*Kale for my bunny rabbit!*

*Mushrooms!* as you pointed at a pallet of onions!

I was glad that half my face was covered by a mask as you also told every young woman you saw, *You are my mummy!*

### 9th October 2020 – Two Hundred Days Since Lockdown Began

The last working day of the week, which you spend with

Nana Roz, has been nicknamed 'Fun Friday'. You tend to have a sleep for her which makes it slightly more fun for Mummy and Daddy. Today, Great-Nana Mave sent you home with two dozen eggs. Omelettes for you for the foreseeable then!

The list of countries we can visit without having to isolate for two weeks on our return is reducing every week. I have booked October half-term, at the end of the month, off work. Desperate to get away, we booked an Air BnB in Riga, Latvia, for a few nights. After a spot of due diligence, this was quickly cancelled when we found out we would have had to self-isolate in the apartment for the duration of our stay!

**11th October 2020**
Twelve months ago, Mummy and I decided to pursue your interest in football and sign you up for pre-school toddler classes with Diddikicks. This morning, I took you for a trial to see if you enjoyed it. Mummy was gutted Covid-19 restrictions meant that only one adult was allowed to go with you.

You thoroughly enjoyed it and the coaches remarked how good you are. So we set up the direct debit for you to attend every week, at an age five years younger than I can remember playing kids' football.

With the girls out for the afternoon, I took you to an Italian restaurant with Grandad, Liam and Darcie. The plan was for you to make your own pizzas, only to find out that was no longer an option due to coronavirus. I struggled to enjoy my meal as you requested to be taken to the toilet seven times!

I sent you to ask for the bill and, instead, the waitress brought over another babyccino for you. Something was lost in translation there!

Chapter 12

# THE THREE-TIER LOCKDOWN SYSTEM

**12ᵗʰ October 2020**

Last week, rumours spread through the media that the Government was considering imposing a tiered lockdown system. Positive cases of Covid-19 have risen on a daily basis since mid-August. The country is now recording an average of 14,000 Covid-19 cases every day.

From 14ᵗʰ October, England will be split into three Covid-19 alert levels – medium, high and very high. Areas on medium alert are able to socialise in groups of six, both indoors and outdoors.

We are in an area on high alert. This means we can no longer mix with members of a different household indoors. The only area of the country on very high alert is the Liverpool city region. There, they cannot mix with anyone outside of their household anywhere. All premises serving alcohol have to be closed completely until further notice.

The alert level is going be reviewed every four weeks and is dependent on the number of positive Covid-19 cases in each area.

There are concerns that hospitals are reaching their capacity. The introduction of the three-tiered system is an attempt to try and protect the NHS throughout the winter, when Covid-19 levels are expected to rise.

There are more people in hospital with Covid-19 today than there were when the country went into lockdown on 23rd March. Such news makes you reflect on the lack of progress we have actually made. When lockdown began, many people thought we would be through the worst of it within twelve weeks. Now, almost seven months later, we have no idea what we might have to prepare ourselves for.

### 14th October 2020

As Grandma and Grandad are in our 'childcare bubble', it is fine for you and Darcie to go to their house on a Wednesday. Due to our area being on high alert, however, it is illegal for your parents to stay for tea.

Each week, you have breakfast at your grandparents' house and then go to the park and have a toasted teacake for 'brunch' in the café. Today, you fed the squirrels nuts.

A daily record of 19,724 positive Covid-19 cases were reported and 137 people sadly passed away. There are more than 4,000 patients in hospitals up and down the country battling coronavirus.

### 15th October 2020

Today marked ten years since your Mummy and I got

together. Grandma picked you up from nursery, and put you to bed, so we could enjoy a quiet meal out.

The Government wants to move our area into the very-high alert level. Our region's mayor wants assurances over how much pay those people forced away from work are going to receive if this happens.

**16th October 2020**
The first thing you asked when you woke up was, *Mummy? Mummy? Where's Grandma?* You thought that she had stayed over at our house!

Your Diddikicks welcome pack arrived. You were so excited to wear the kit with your name and a number '2' on the back that you went to bed dressed in it!

The Government moved Lancashire into the high alert level, also referred to as Tier 3. This meant that Mummy and I changed the venue of our overnight stay tomorrow to Yorkshire, as they are still in Tier 2. Being in lockdown has started to test our organisational skills!

**17th October 2020**
Swimming lessons started back up again for the first time since March. The significant difference was that you had to go in the pool on your own. This was a surprise to Mummy as you were abruptly snatched from her at the door which left her to return to the car in floods of tears. You greeted her with a smile as you waited in line to be collected at the fire exit on the way out so next week should be a touch easier for her.

Mummy and I went away for the night so you stayed with Nana Roz and *Nana* James. We had to check into every hospitality establishment using the NHS Test and

Trace app and confirm that we lived together. Such is now the norm on a Covid-19 night out.

**20th October 2020**
Yesterday, Wales announced that they are going into full lockdown for seventeen days from Friday.

Today, the inevitable happened as the Government forced our region into Tier 3, with effect from 23rd October. The last hope of getting away for half-term was gone in an instant as we are now not allowed to leave the area. Technically, there are actually four tiers with the highest one meaning 'stay at home'.

Hallowe'en season got underway at nursery. We might be in for a week of trepidation as you were physically sick when thinking about witches!

**21st October 2020**
You and Darcie did not enjoy the most amicable start to the day at Grandma and Grandad's. You hit her in the face with a Lion King teddy because you wanted her *bun buns* soft toy. For the first time ever, she hit you back! Good girl!

There were 26,688 cases of Covid-19 reported in the country today. Worryingly, this is the highest daily total recorded so far.

Spain became the first country in Europe to record one million positive cases of coronavirus.

*Chapter 13*

# TIER THREE, FOR FOUR WEEKS AT LEAST

**23rd October 2020**
As of 12.01am today, our region moved into Tier 3. This is the highest alert level aside from simply being asked to stay at home. We can now be fined if we mix with anyone from another household – indoors or outdoors – apart from our 'support bubbles'. This means that your grandparents can still look after you as normal.

You went to see Great-Nana Mave with Nana Roz. This is also allowed as Nana Roz does things to care for Great-Nana Mave, such as take her shopping and collect prescriptions for her.

You rolled around Great-Nana Mave's living room floor with your dumper truck and a set of dice. You argued that there is a face on a dice with seven dots on it!

## 24th October 2020

It is difficult to report anything of note when you go swimming because Mummy cannot go in with you!

When I got home you asked me, *Why do you play golf in the rain?!* You try and do what you can to get out when you are in Tier 3, Little Man!

After being scared to go to nursery earlier in the week, you are now warming to Hallowe'en. You went with Mummy to buy a costume, pumpkin and decorations from the supermarket. You loved carving the pumpkin at home and referred to the witches and vampires bunting, after much brainwashing from Mummy, as *cute*.

## 27th October 2020

Whilst there's guidance from the Government against travelling in and out of Tier 3 areas, technically, it is not illegal. Life in lockdown is difficult and the monotony of home, against a backdrop of the unknown, creates a yearning for the freedom that we once naturally enjoyed. So, we decided to take a few days away on the North East Yorkshire coast.

You slept the majority of the drive to Staithes where we had lunch. You are very good at entertaining yourself in restaurants. Invariably, you choose to create scenarios with your dinosaurs, making them 'talk' to one another in funny little voices.

After lunch, we took a walk down to the beach and put some seaweed in a bucket for the crabs you hoped to catch. You wanted to hang around and build some sandcastles but the wind and drizzle did not exactly lend itself to such a serene activity.

Our *holiday house* in Whitby was a second-floor, one bedroom flat. You chose to sleep on the bed near the window as you wanted to look at the church.

On the way into the town centre you enjoyed looking at all the Hallowe'en decorations in the windows. *What's the pumpkin doing? What's that witch doing there? What's that skeleton doing?*

## 28th October 2020

After breakfast we walked down to 'Kiddies Corner' on the harbour, which is popular for crabbing. The tide was not fully in but the one crab we caught was enough to keep you happy.

We stopped off for a coffee in a café that was also a bookshop. Life became very difficult for you as you wanted to buy *Tyrannosaurus Drip*, a book you already had at home. After twenty minutes of tears, snot, glazed eyes, shouting, arm-waving, rolling around on the floor and a short walk around the block to calm you down, you were content with buying *The Girl and the Dinosaur*. This was a lovely book that I read to you twice as you sipped on your babyccino.

We drove to Saltburn-by-the-Sea for lunch. We then took a steep walk down to the pier. The social anxiety perpetuated by Covid-19 means that interactions with strangers are a rarity. Mummy and I were therefore taken aback when a couple stopped to ask if we would like them to take a photograph of the three of us using Mummy's mobile phone.

There was a long queue to get into the games arcade. For all our efforts on the 2p machines, a basketball game and one involving balls and tubes you collected enough tickets to win a solitary, sticky crab. When we got back to the car, we homed this blob of goo above my steering wheel on the dashboard.

Despite Whitby being in Tier 1, the lowest alert level, it is impossible to escape the impact Covid-19 continues to have on daily life. Leaving 'Kiddies Corner' this morning, I asked a young family if they would like to take our crab off us. This simple, friendly gesture was abruptly declined. As far as we were aware, Covid-19 had yet to infect the crustacean population!

In the coffee shop, you walked towards a man who was sat down and he blurted, 'Uh! Go away!' as though you were a living, breathing personification of coronavirus.

Obliviously walking back across the swing bridge in Whitby, another man barked that we were on the wrong side of the one-way system. Your acts of innocence largely contrast against the broader anxiety, paranoia and fear that has become ingrained into certain sections of society.

**29th October 2020**
The road from Whitby to Scarborough winds and dips across the North Yorkshire moors. *Whoa!* you cried as my driving caused a funny sensation for you down below. *That tickled my willy!* you giggled.

*Rain, rain, go away! Come again another day!* you sang as we walked into the wind and drizzle round Scarborough's seafront. We sheltered from the wet weather in a games arcade and you are becoming quite fond of gambling 2p coins away.

After visiting a souvenir shop you complained that the double-decker bus you bought *doesn't drive very well.*

This led to one of your now-frequent tantrums which only stopped when you started eating your chippy lunch in the car.

Back in Whitby, you remembered the way we walked down to the harbour was the same way we walked back to our Air BnB last night – *along the 'clibbers'* (cobbles). You have quite an impressive memory for a two-year-old.

After you declined the offer of a boat trip we walked the 199 steps to Whitby Abbey (the *Vampire's Castle*). You made a good effort of counting the steps, improvising when you were not sure how to carry on. *Twenty-seven, twenty-eight, twenty-nine, twenty-ten, twenty eleven!*

There is a strong Hallowe'en theme in Whitby and you were scared of a man dressed up in the doorway of a shop. You audibly made the same feelings known about a woman in the doorway of the next shop. What tickled Mummy and I was that this poor lady was kitted out in her own clothes!

Some of the things you say in your broad, northern accent have me and Mummy in stitches. *That's massive!* you shouted, pointing at a spider covering the gable end of a pub and, *Size of it!* at another large arachnid in the display of a fishmonger's shop!

### 30th October 2020

Waking to dangerously high levels of energy, you ran around the flat as Mummy and I packed up to leave. Your tornado impression was abruptly jolted when you ran into a wall.

The weather was wet and grim once again. We had a drive to Robin Hood's Bay, famous for fossils. Intent on uncovering a whole diplodocus skeleton, you had to settle for a handful of live hermit crabs!

Back in Whitby, we bribed you on to the *happy boat* after a lunch of fish and chips. Despite being insistent you did not want to go on a boat ride, you did not shut up for the twenty minute journey out to sea and back. On returning to the harbour, you remarked, *The water is flat now!* in contrast to the *wobbly water* out at sea. Those waiting for the next boat trip were then treated to you relieving yourself off the end of the jetty. After a picture with me under the famous Whitby Whale Bone Arch, we set off home.

Before bed, Mummy asked you to reflect on what you had enjoyed most about the last few days. Your answer, after all we had done, was, *Playing with my dinosaurs.*

### 31st October 2020
Hallowe'en.

You gave me a sound piece of advice as I left the house to play golf in the rain, *Wear your coat.*

We went to Grandma and Grandad's in the afternoon. You were dressed in a spider costume, telling us how much you were going to scare everyone. This was until you were fearful of Grandma with her witch's hat and broomstick!

Grandma was more excited than you and Darcie so off you went trick or treating down the street before dark. You visited two of the neighbours and got your plastic orange cauldrons filled with goodies. Remembering the importance of a balanced diet you asked Trevor and Diane at number 7 if they had any bananas!

At 6.30pm the prime minister announced to the nation

that England will go back into full lockdown – Tier 4 – on Thursday 5th November at 12.01am. This means that all pubs, bars, restaurants and non-essential businesses will close. Nurseries, schools, colleges and universities are able to remain open.

The Government claims that this is absolutely necessary to prevent the spread of Covid-19. Alarmingly, the data warns that if these measures are not taken then the number of deaths in the next month will be double what they were back in April.

As we approach Christmas, families up and down the country are hoping that it can be fully enjoyed after a year of isolation and separation from loved ones. As is becoming depressingly apparent throughout this pandemic, there are certainly no guarantees.

### 4th November 2020

Liam and Emma took Darcie to Chester Zoo and Cheshire Oaks before everything has to close tomorrow. Making the most of what you are allowed to do, before venturing into a period of the unknown, has become the norm for families up and down the country.

Grandma went to work as she has to close the salon for at least four weeks tomorrow. We are now standing on the edge of another full, national lockdown.

You spent the morning with Grandad and were a fantastic help as he attempted to get some jobs done, sweeping leaves and 'washing' his car with your water pistol.

25,177 people tested positive for Covid-19 today and 492 people passed away.

Chapter 14

# LOCKDOWN 2.0: ATTEMPTING TO RESCUE CHRISTMAS

**5th November 2020**

'Remember, remember the fifth of November. Gunpowder, treason and plot'.

This year, there will be no mass gatherings, or any gatherings at all, for Bonfire Night. It will be remembered as the day England went into Lockdown 2.0, as it is being called. This did not stop people setting fireworks off from their gardens. The noise excited you and your voice was almost as loud as the bangs.

You helped set Quartz's cage up in the kitchen as we wanted to bring him in from the clatter outside. You were telling him to get in his cage and go to sleep. A touch hypocritical when sleeping on demand is not something you ever do!

## 7th November 2020

There was no swimming for you and no golf for me as we adjusted to Lockdown 2.0.

The warm and sunny weather gave us the opportunity to go up to the reservoirs. The last time we were here in May you moaned that your balance bike was *too 'wobbedy'* (wobbly). Today you rode around without a fuss.

On the way back up the hill, you had me climbing the steep, grassy banks with you. Either you had no concept of danger or thought that I was a mountaineer, as you wanted to climb the vertical, rock faces that jutted out at the top!

## 8th November 2020

The cyclical nature of living through this pandemic is made all the more glaring now that we are back trying to entertain you at home. The optimism of the spring is absent as we face a dark winter in lockdown.

What else better to do when it is cold and raining outside than buy a few newspapers and make a papier-mâché volcano? The kitchen floor was a mess with flour, water, PVA glue and strips of newspaper scattered around. You kept asking when the volcano was going to *'rupt* (erupt) and enquired, *Where's the lava?* Once you realised that there was not a magma reservoir under our house, you got bored and played with a whisk in the sink.

## 9th November 2020

We certainly did not ask for the working week to start at 5.30am after you wet the bed for the second night running. Yesterday, you woke up at a similar time in tears, crying, *I don't want to eat duck!* Whatever that means!

The pharmaceutical company, Pfizer, announced that they have developed a Covid-19 vaccine which is 90% efficient. This is a major breakthrough. Especially considering that scientists predicted any vaccine made at this stage would only work in half of cases. The Government is hoping to roll this out in early December.

**10$^{th}$ November 2020**
You left the house with a warning to listen at nursery ringing in your ears. The consequences? No television or time on your tablet this evening. Being removed from 'Relax Kids' at nursery, for not being very relaxed, meant that the sanctions had to be upheld.

You are mastering the art of distraction when having to own up to your behaviour. Your response when I asked you why you had not been listening was, *Oh look! A spider web!*

Mummy's teaching assistant was sent home yesterday with suspected Covid-19. Today, the test returned a negative result which means Mummy and the rest of her class do not have to self-isolate for two weeks.

Nana Roz has been moved to work on a Covid-19 ward in hospital due to the usual staff being off sick with the virus. Therefore, we made the decision for you not to see her on Friday this week.

**11$^{th}$ November 2020**
*We're in lockdown. Why we in lockdown?*
'Because we need to slow down the virus, Noah'.
*'Cos the virus running very fast?!* you innocently enquired.

**15th November 2020**

We wrapped up, sporting our new wellies, and retraced our footsteps from the first lockdown in the spring. Walking down into the dell, Mummy slipped and fell. You turned around, spotted her on the deck and candidly asked, *What you doing down there?*

We waded up the stream near the 'Gruffalo's Cave' and your wellies and waterproof pants were not enough to stop your boots flooding with water. That, and slipping and hurting your little finger, made the walk up and out of the dell less enjoyable.

A funny mannerism you have developed, which started in Whitby, is to randomly shout, *Hey! Double-yoo!* The only explanation Mummy and I have thought of is that you have confused the letter 'W' with the word, 'you'. How? We have no idea!

After seeing a man fishing in the pond, you stopped at every puddle and dipped a stick in. You put a 'whale' and a 'shark' in an imaginary bucket and carried a 'crab' in your other hand all the way home. Living life as a toddler, oblivious to the terrifying events going on across the globe, is definitely the place to be!

**16th November 2020**

Today, Mummy and I celebrated eight years of living in our house. This time next year we will hopefully have moved into our new house which is being rebuilt.

Moderna, another pharmaceutical company, have also produced a vaccine for Covid-19. They claim that this one is even more effective than the one Pfizer reported last week.

**18th November 2020**

Last Friday when you went to Grandma and Grandad's, you wore your Pudsey Bear jumper for Children in Need. You told people that your Mummy had bought this for you so that other children's *mummies and daddies could have pennies*. Today, you decided that you wanted to wear it again.

The Government are considering allowing households to mix for five days over Christmas. However, to counteract the inevitable transmission of the virus this would result in, we would need to remain in lockdown for twenty-five days either side of 25th December.

There were 529 deaths from the virus today. A total of 53,274 people have now died from Covid-19. The number of positive test results shows no sign of abating with a further 19,609 today.

**21st November 2020**

All week you have been really good at going to the toilet when you should. This morning, you wet yourself twice before we left the house. Another 'accident', along with a traditional supermarket tantrum over some chocolate buttons, led to lots of shouting and tears.

We drove to Blackpool and walked down the promenade from the Pleasure Beach to the Tower. You pressed your nose up against the glass at the 'Sandcastle' waterpark and South Pier arcades, not understanding why everything was closed.

A man wearing a bandana served us at the chippy. *Look! A pirate!* you shouted at him over the counter.

The plan had been to walk back to the car under the

illuminations. For some ridiculous reason, Mummy and I had not stopped to think that they had been cancelled this year because of the pandemic.

As the sun set into the Irish Sea, I said, 'Look, Noah. The sun is falling into the sea.' You responded nonchalantly, *No, Daddy… it is setting.* I will give trying to be magical a rest then shall I?!

### 23rd November 2020

Throughout the pandemic, it has become clear that the only way out is through mass vaccination. Oxford University/AstraZeneca have produced a Covid-19 vaccine which has been 90% effective in clinical trials. The prime minister hopes that the 'vast majority' of vulnerable people will have been vaccinated against Covid-19 by Easter 2021.

When lockdown ends on 2nd December, the country will return to the tiered system which preceded it. In Tier 1 areas, 4,000 people will be able to attend football matches.

For us, not much will change as we will more than likely revert to being in Tier 3.

### 24th November 2020

The Government announced its plans to enable families to spend Christmas together. Apparently, people will be able to form a 'bubble' of up to three households. On both sides of our family, there are eight households so it is anyone's guess how we are going to work things out!

607 people died from Covid-19. This is the highest daily total since May.

### 25th November 2020

Mummy has decided to restrict unnecessary contact with others as the staffing situation in her school is dire. This includes picking you up from childcare.

Liam and Emma booked to go to Dubai for a week on your birthday. At the start of the month, the United Arab Emirates was removed from the list of countries where you have to quarantine on your return.

The highest total of daily deaths since May was topped for a second consecutive day. Sadly, 696 people died today.

Diego Maradona, widely regarded as the greatest footballer to have ever lived, died of a heart attack aged sixty. Such was the outpouring of grief in his home country of Argentina, that the president declared three days of national mourning.

### 26th November 2020

Reflecting on the impact Covid-19 and the pandemic has had on our household, we have been relatively lucky. None of us has been ill from the virus. We have not lost any earnings as a consequence of the pandemic. No one has had to self-isolate after a positive Covid-19 test and we have not been contacted by the 'Track and Trace' app to inform us that we have been in close contact with someone subsequently testing positive for Covid-19.

Today, all that could change. Mummy had to pick you up from nursery because you had a temperature, one of the symptoms of Covid-19. I left work to meet you and Mummy outside the testing centre that had been erected on a car park outside the Town Hall.

To attend the testing centre, you had to book

appointments and arrive at a specific time. We checked into the sprawling white medical tent where we were assigned a booth by a woman wearing a mask. Mummy and I had to swab both nostrils, whereas you only needed to have one swabbed. You were very brave, sitting on my knee as Mummy stuck the thin, plastic implement up your nose. You said that it tickled and coughed as the swab hit the top of your nasal cavity.

This went as well as we could have expected and you were very happy with the three stickers you got for being a *big boy*. Leaving the tent you announced, *All the coronavirus has been scraped out of my nose!*

Until we know the results we now have to stay at home. If any one of us tests positive then we face the prospect of the next two weeks in self-isolation. If it transpires that you have coronavirus, you will have to spend your third birthday in quarantine.

### 27th November 2020

By mid-morning, one by one, our negative tests results had come through on our mobile phones. This meant that Mummy and I could go back to work and you went to Grandma and Grandad's for the day.

Living in limbo is a strange feeling. We had mentally prepared ourselves for the possibility of two weeks at home. Now, we are back to 'normal' until we hit another bump on this road the pandemic is laying out for us.

### 28th November 2020 – 250 Days Since Lockdown Began

It has been the strangest year of our lives so far. Keeping up with the oddities of lockdown, we put our Christmas tree up in November for the first time ever. You decorated a little tree which you put on your table in the kitchen and then pottered around the front room pretending to be helpful.

We got into the Christmas spirit, wearing Christmas-themed headbands and listening to Christmas songs. You and I left Mummy to finish decorating the tree in peace and went shopping for your birthday cake. You insisted on wearing your sparkly Rudolph antlers for the trip, which attracted a few complimentary glances!

Chapter 15

# A COVID-19 CHRISTMAS

**1st December 2020**
For the first time, you have got an awareness of Christmas, its meaning and what there is to look forward to on Christmas Day.

I was happy to let Mummy take the credit for introducing 'Elf on the Shelf' to our household, where a 'funny' elf pops up in a different place each day. We steered clear of calling him a 'naughty' elf as Mummy did not want to provide you with any unnecessary encouragement!

This morning, you woke up to the elf sat on the chest of drawers in your bedroom. He was holding a letter from Father Christmas, informing you that his elf was going to be watching you and reporting back whether you had been using your 'listening ears'.

When you got home from nursery you told us that you were off to *open 'umber two* on your advent calendar. Not until tomorrow, Little Man!

**2nd December 2020**
Overnight, the four-week national lockdown ended and the country slipped back into the tiered system that had preceded it. We are in Tier 3 which means that we cannot mix with people from other households indoors and pubs and restaurants remain closed. Our tier will be reviewed on a fortnightly basis.

In Tier 1 and 2 areas, football fans were allowed to attend matches inside stadiums for the first time since March.

**4th December 2020**
Our country became the first in the world to roll out a national Covid-19 vaccination programme. The jabs will be provided to the most vulnerable in society first as well as to people who work on the front line in health and social care professions.

**5th December 2020**
Your third birthday, or *'umber three* as you referred to your new age.

Three years since you arrived into our lives and changed them forever. The constraints of the pandemic have meant that we have been able to observe your transformation from very close quarters. No longer a baby, or even a toddler, but a clever, inquisitive, funny, happy, cheeky, loving and mischievous little boy!

Before swimming, you opened some presents and walked around the house singing, *Happy birthday to me!* You recorded a birthday message for your friend Ben, who was four today, the main lyrics being, *Happy birthday to us!*

We had booked to go on a 'Santa Express' train ride

but, you guessed it, Covid-19 had it cancelled. Instead, we went to a drive-thru Santa's grotto in the city centre. Even if you had enjoyed it, it would still have been the worst festive experience of our lives!

Picture a large empty car park, the 'road' marked out by cones. A metal shack, under which Father Christmas sat, was where you received your present through the car window. At the end of this magical adventure, we parked the car up and fed 'Rudolph', a live reindeer in a makeshift stable, some moss. This was a brief highlight until Father Christmas joined us, given you were petrified of him.

Santa had a few elves, who would not have looked out of place in a Christmas-themed adult entertainment video. The authenticity of the elves' plunged to new depths when one of them referred to her boss as 'Santa Christmas'!

You were not alone when you cried, *I want to go home now!* We saw the funny side of this appalling attempt at trying to keep the magic of Christmas alive in the midst of a pandemic. Back home, you rattled through opening the rest of your presents one by one.

On the whole, we all enjoyed a great day and it was lovely to see you wrapped up in the excitement of your third birthday. Apart from meeting the big man himself. *Don't want to see Father Christmas again!* you told Mummy as she kissed you goodnight.

## 6th December 2020

Yesterday, at the grotto, Father Christmas should have called my mobile phone to talk to you. In keeping with the dreadful experience, he forgot! So, I arranged for him to call as you were having your breakfast. His popularity with you had not risen overnight and you were equally as frightened of his voice on loudspeaker as you were of him in person. Your face was a contorted mixture of panic and fear as he asked what you wanted for Christmas.

Eventually, he coaxed your Christmas list out of you. A car garage, a blue car and a yo-yo. We wondered where the idea for you to want a toy that was popular in the '70s and '80s came from!

## 8th December 2020

A ninety-year-old grandmother from Coventry became the first person in the world to receive the Pfizer Covid-19 vaccine. This kicked off the largest vaccination programme in the history of the NHS.

*What's that?* you asked, grabbing hold of a stainless-steel spirit measure.

'That's for measuring Mummy's gin', I answered.

*Like this?* you enquired, holding it across the bottom of your chin.

## 13th December 2020

You forgot to use your 'listening ears' at Diddikicks but this did not deter the coaches from being taken in by your charm. It is amazing how much children love stickers and you proudly puffed out your chest walking back to my car with one stuck to your shirt.

Grandma and Grandad went for Covid-19 tests two days ago as Grandad had worked in someone's house who subsequently tested positive for the virus. Both tests came back negative. A less favourable result would have seen them stuck at home alone for Christmas.

The biggest, and most exciting, news of the year in our household arrived just before tea. Mummy found out that she was pregnant! It could prove to be very difficult news to keep quiet over the Christmas period, lockdown or not.

As Mummy and I discussed this news in hushed voices, we noticed that you had been very quiet. We looked around at the kitchen table where you had fallen asleep on your plate, corn-on-the-cob in hand. It was 5.40pm!

**16th December 2020**
The elf made his way to the top of your Christmas tree overnight, which you were not too happy about when you saw him this morning.

I took the morning off work and took you to see Old Trafford for the first time. As we drove through the drizzle you casually asked, *Is coronavirus still here? Has the rain washed it away?* A heart-warming insight into the mind of a three-year-old.

Before you were born, I spent many afternoons and evenings on the damp streets of Stretford, selling the fanzine *United We Stand*. So, it was only apt that you posed for a photograph in my favourite selling spot on Sir Matt Busby Way, holding a copy of the mag aloft.

Despite Bruno Fernandes being your favourite player, you wanted Donny van de Beek's name printed on the back of your shirt in the megastore. On the way out, you asked a steward if the stadium was open and declared, *I will score a goal!* We walked a lap of Old Trafford with your new ball tucked under your arm. Your boots and socks were soaked by the end from jumping in every puddle you came across.

Mummy worked from home in the afternoon which brought back memories for her of trying to work and parent you at the same time.

612 individuals passed away from Covid-19 today. The total now stands at 65,440. Frighteningly, this is nearly enough people to fill Old Trafford.

### 17th December 2020

Yesterday, London, Essex and Hertfordshire were placed into Tier 4, where they will remain for Christmas.

Today, the Government decided to keep our region in Tier 4 which means that is where we will spend the festive period.

It was Christmas jumper day for you at nursery. Your last day there in what has been a very strange and fractured year.

It was also Mummy's last day at work until the New Year. She would have ordinarily celebrated at home with a glass of mulled wine. Not now that she is carrying your baby sibling!

### 19th December 2020

*Don't get ready!* you shouted at me as I was putting on my clothes for golf. Trying to guilt-trip either me or Mummy is something you are becoming quite good at.

Games of golf regularly throw up strange things. Today, on the eleventh hole, a crow swooped down, picked my playing partner's ball up in its beak, and flew away!

Retelling this story when I got home preoccupied you for the afternoon. You constantly asked, *Why? I don't like that crow!* and *Naughty crow!*

We have become used to waiting for the announcements from the Prime Minister, Boris Johnson, throughout the pandemic. Often, as you tune into the television broadcasts, it is only for confirmation of what we already know.

At teatime, Boris more or less made the decision to cancel Christmas. A new variant of Covid-19 is spreading quickly across parts of the country. London, as well as parts of the east and south east of England, moved into Tier 4 for Christmas. This means that they are not allowed to mix with anyone from outside of their own household.

For the rest of the country, the five-day window allowing people to mix with up to three households has now been reduced to Christmas Day only.

## 22nd December 2020

*Boys have willies. Girls don't have willies. Darcie has a nunny. Do you have a nunny, Mummy?* That's what Mummy had to listen to as you both went for a walk round the lake.

It was a cold day and you complained that your hands were stinging. Despite the winter weather, some cafés were only serving food and drink outside. You were reluctant to sit on the only bench available because it was covered in blotches of bird poo. Mummy eventually persuaded you to sit down until a seagull relieved itself on the shoulder of your coat!

## 23rd December 2020

I finished work yesterday so today marked the start of a full week at home as a family. You came with me to do a round of errands. Your behaviour went from the sublime to the ridiculous, as a three-year-old's brain often dictates!

You were helpful at the tip and sat nicely in my work's office eating a cupcake. At the supermarket you screamed, *Put me down! I'm not a baby!* as I tried to get you to sit in the trolley. At Grandma and Grandad's house, you refused to get out and help me put a few things in the car.

Back at home, you did help me wash the table down outside. In a moment of comical karma, the wind flicked the table round which knocked a bucket of soapy water into your face!

Preparing for Christmas Day, we pushed the sofas back to make more room in the centre of the lounge. Inevitably, the added space gave you the licence to charge around!

Two more sleeps until your 'best mate' comes.

### 24th December 2020
Christmas Eve.

You woke up at 5am and tried to get in our bed, only to be sent back. In your head, by the time you had got up at the normal time of 7am you had completed the two sleeps required before Christmas Day. Nice try, Little Man!

I took you to the park to meet Parry, his son Ben, Birchy and his children Matilda and Theo. These are close friends who we have hardly seen all year because of the pandemic. It is sad because you would have all been a lot closer were it not for the disruption caused to our lives. It was a bitterly cold day and you kept asking me to blow on your hands to warm them up!

In the afternoon, we spent some time in the back garden at Grandma and Grandad's with Liam, Emma and Darcie. You and I wore matching Christmas jumpers. At

2.30pm we had a surprise visit from Father Christmas. Thankfully, you loved seeing him, which was a relief given the frights he has previously given you!

Darcie asked, *Where's Rudolph?* and you both sang Santa Christmas songs. Grandma asked whether Father Christmas would like a drink, meaning champagne, and you piped up, *Would you like some blackcurrant?* You both had a great time seeing him and waved him off from the back gate.

At home, the elf had left the top of our Christmas tree to return to the North Pole. His parting gift was a Christmas Eve box which contained Christmas pyjamas for the three of us and some books for you.

Before going to bed, you left Father Christmas a mince pie and some whisky, as well as a carrot for Rudolph, on the fireplace. Quartz had a good go at tucking into that before Mummy and I went to bed!

### 25th December 2020
Christmas Day.

Walking into the front room from the bottom of the stairs, you were more interested in whether the mince pie, whisky and carrot had gone than you were in the pile of presents under the tree. Despite seeming to understand how Christmas Day worked in the build-up to today, you were still overwhelmed by everything.

*Open the curtains… let me see the snow!* Someone had obviously bought into the imagery portrayed in so many Christmas films.

*Oh look! Santa dropped some presents!* you cried, not realising that they were for you.

Each present you opened was followed by a sharp intake of breath, an excited squeal or a curious *Oooooooh!* Your attention was fixated on the most recent present you had opened, with you forgetting that there were more to get through.

Mummy's construction of your new car garage took a lot longer than it should have done because you were either moving the parts away or trying to ride the cars in an out before it was built.

It did snow in other parts of the country today, making it officially a white Christmas. Shortly after lunch a few snowflakes fell on our garden.

For as long as I can remember, we did not meet our family in the pub at lunch-time on Christmas Day. Whilst trivial in the grand scheme of things, it does hit home when customs that have been taken for granted are removed. Having said that, given the way this year has gone, it hardly came as a surprise.

The lockdown rules dictated that three households could gather together for Christmas Day. Technically, these were broken as we had Stevie and Simon, Great-Nana Mave and Great-Nana Anne and Great-Grandad Mike for Christmas Dinner. In the lead-up, many hours had been dedicated to debating what was best for our family on Christmas Day. Some of these conversations were then rendered meaningless as the Government changed the rules. Not having the aforementioned three households for dinner would have meant someone would have had to spend Christmas Day alone. An impossible choice in what has turned out to be an impossible year.

As you sat down at the table for dinner, you clutched

a jar from the centre and asked blunty, *Anyone want any cranberry?*

You really enjoyed the chocolate pudding that Stevie and Simon had made and, obviously, asked for more!

After such a difficult year, it was so nice to have all three of your great-grandparents round at out house to celebrate. Despite the day being far from normal, everyone had a great time.

### 28th December 2020

The Government announced that secondary school pupils, apart from those in Year 11 studying for their GCSEs, will not return as planned on 4th January 2021.

Hospitals in the UK are now treating more people for Covid-19 than they were at the peak of infections back in April. A total of 41,385 positive Covid-19 test results were recorded today. This is the highest daily increase since the pandemic began and perhaps an indication that we were not the only ones to break the rules on Christmas Day.

The number of people who have died from the virus in the UK now stands at 71,109.

### 29th December 2020

We woke up to a dusting of snow on our street. *Why?* was your ever-so-common response, as you peered out of the bedroom window. Perhaps because it is cold, Little Man!

Our promise to take you to Dino Falls Adventure Golf perished when you tripped and split your head on the corner of the wall near the porch door. *Don't want my head to hurt! Don't want a plaster!* you wailed in the back of my car on the way to the accident and emergency department. On first inspection, you were going to need a bit more than a plaster!

Due to Covid-19, only one of us was allowed to accompany you into the hospital. Mummy had responded a little calmer than me to the whole event so she took you in for your forehead to be glued and *train track* (butterfly) stitches to be applied across your wound. You were a very brave boy, although you did not think so yourself, muttering to the nurse, *I have had a big bump. I were sad.*

### 30th December 2020

The snow had fallen thicker on the ground so, with me at work, you went to the park with Mummy. You were not able to make snowballs because the snow kept sticking to your gloves. Mummy ended up making the snowballs to pass to you, only for you to then throw them at her!

You cannot get your hair wet for another four days but you are more than happy to wear *Mummy's special hat* (shower cap) for bathtime.

The Government moved our region into Tier 4, which now means no mixing with anyone outside of our household and that all non-essential shops must close. Approximately 40% of the country is now living in Tier 4.

The UK recorded 50,023 positive cases of Covid-19 today, with 981 people losing their lives. This is the highest daily death total since 24th April and the virus shows no signs of slowing down as the year comes to a close.

### 31ˢᵗ December 2020

New Year's Eve. A cold and foggy day. You and Mummy went for a walk around the lake. Mummy sent me a picture of you lying under your bike on the dirt track, caked in mud from the waist down. This was quickly followed by one of you happily eating chips from a tray with your hands!

Only Stevie and Simon know that Mummy is having a baby so they looked after you for a few hours whilst Mummy attended an appointment with the midwife.

Back at home, Mummy read you your final bedtime story of the weirdest year in living memory. As I tucked you in, you counted down the four fingers I had held up to signify the number of people who will be our family this time next year. *Mummy, Daddy, Noah, Baby*.

Mummy, sober, and I stayed in on our own on New Year's Eve for the first time ever. It was very emotional watching the fireworks illuminate the sky over the town from our bedroom window. As the colours exploded through the darkness, we reflected on 2020. A year that will inarguably go down as one of the strangest, most difficult and heart-wrenching for millions of people across the globe. A year in which a virus spread indiscriminately around the world, turned cities into vacuums and changed people's lives, in some cases, forever.

As a family in 2021, we have so much to look forward to. We have a baby and, maybe, a house move on the way. As the vaccine is rolled out nationally, we will hopefully go on holiday abroad for the first time since August 2019.

Over the last nine months we have witnessed you grow and change, physically and emotionally, in so many ways. Like thousands of other children, your social development has taken a hit at times. Through it all, we are so proud of you and your absorbing, energising, loving character.

Happy New Year, Little Man!

**1st January 2021**
New Year's Day. Vomiting twice during the night were your first two acts of 2021.

Getting you to do as you are asked, when you are asked, is one of parenthood's fresh challenges for us. When I paused the tablet for you, after you failed to do it the first three times I politely requested, you had a meltdown which put paid to our plan to go for a walk at lunchtime. We opted for a drive instead and the fact you slept for two hours hinted that you were perhaps coming down with something.

New Year's Day was another family occasion dissolved by the pandemic as we spent it at home as a trio. We used up the last of the Christmas crackers and you ended up spending an inordinate amount of time trying to find a frog that you lost out of one! The first day of 2021 ended with it still missing.

**2nd January 2021**
Great-Nana Anne's seventy-seventh birthday.

It was time to rid ourselves of Christmas in our house and take the tree and decorations down. As usual, you participated in your own unique way. This involved you polishing your toys with antibacterial wipes!

As I put the tree where it belonged, you had your first experience of being in the attic, declaring, *I love it in the loft!* You did not stick around for too long after I told you it was where the spiders lived!

### 3rd **January 2021**

We finally made it to Dino Falls Adventure Golf, after our aborted attempt last week. You told me, *I'm going to beat you, I'm very fast!* Since when has golf been a matter of raw speed, Little Man?!

Your strategy was questionable as you frequently attempted the most difficult route to the hole. To your credit, you did manage a hole-in-one on your favourite hole, where you had to putt the ball into a stream which then carried it towards its destination.

Today was the sixth in a row where more than 50,000 positive Covid-19 tests results were recorded. Over 75,000 people have now died from the virus in the UK.

Chapter 16

# LOCKDOWN 3.0

**4th January 2021**
Thousands of schools across the country remained closed after the Christmas holidays. Mummy went back to work although a number of parents of children at her school refused to send their children in.

The new variant of Covid-19 is causing nationwide chaos. Scientists report that it spreads much more quickly than the original strain. The highest number of daily cases of Covid-19 since the pandemic began were recorded, a staggering 58,784.

At 8pm, Boris Johnson announced that the whole country has to go into Tier 4 lockdown from 6th January. The message is 'Stay at Home', unless it is absolutely necessary to leave your house. This means that schools will be forced to shut until after the February half-term, at least.

What was I saying about Happy New Year?

**6th January 2021**

Lockdown 3.0 legally came into force. There is no guarantee when this latest lockdown will end. The regulations are poised to remain in place until the end of March.

Yesterday, the number of identified Covid-19 cases topped 60,000 for the very first time.

Elite sport is allowed to continue, which was not the case during the first lockdown last year. I wish it had been forced to stop, with Manchester City knocking United out of the League Cup at the semi-final stage for the second season running.

**8th January 2021**

All international travellers will soon have to produce a negative Covid-19 test before entering the country. Why this is only being put into place 291 days into the pandemic is anyone's guess!

Ominously, the records for the number of Covid-19 cases and deaths from the virus tumble on an almost daily basis. It certainly feels as though this situation will worsen before it improves. 1,325 deaths and 68,053 positive cases today. Devastating.

**9th January 2021**

With the holiday season over, weekends are beginning to feel very much like they did in the first lockdown. Unlike last spring, the days are much wetter and colder.

With literally nothing else to do we went for a walk down into the dell and over the moors. We managed to stop you from going into the icy stream but not from falling over about three dozen times.

Once we were home and had warmed up, you painted the papier-mâché volcano we built over two months ago!

Nana Roz and James became the first people in our family to receive the Covid-19 vaccine.

**13th January 2021**
Darcie's feeling the effects of this third lockdown, telling Uncle Liam and Auntie Emma, *I have not seen Noah for hours and hours!* This situation takes its toll on intelligent, well-informed, understanding adults. Such statements highlight how it must feel for children lacking the same comprehension.

Great-Nana Mave received the Covid-19 vaccine yesterday.

A record 1,564 people died today, taking the total number of deaths in the country to 84,767. The gravity of the pandemic is weighing heavily on the nation. The severity of what we are living through feels starker as each dark day passes.

**14th January 2021**
Seeing as you got up shortly after 6am, I decided to join you and put the first day of England's first Test match in Sri Lanka on the television. They were playing at the picturesque ground in Galle, surrounded on three sides by the Pacific Ocean, beneath the Dutch Fort. Mummy and I watched Sri Lanka play Pakistan in a Test match there in August 2014. You could not quite get your head around the fact it was daytime in Galle and how the players stopped play for lunch before you had eaten your breakfast!

A new coronavirus variant in Brazil has meant that the Government is stopping all flights into the country from South America, Portugal and Cape Verde from 4am tomorrow morning.

### 15th January 2021

Due to Nana Roz coming into close contact with lots of people infected with Covid-19 in hospital this week, we decided against her looking after you today. Mummy took care of you at home, which was a tough balancing act as she still had to work. She tried to keep you occupied, feeding you snacks and cleaning up after you whilst she attended meetings online.

New terminology continues to seep into everyday language. The R rate is something that we have become accustomed to hearing about. This is a number used to describe the transmissibility of a virus. Basically, how many people an infected person is likely to spread the virus to. If the R rate remains above 1, then it means the virus is not slowing down. The Government informed us that the R rate in the UK is between 1.2 and 1.5.

More positively, the peak of infections and deaths is thought to have passed. However, the height of the number of people in hospital with Covid-19 is not likely to be reached for another seven to ten days.

### 18th January 2021

Over four million people have now received their first Covid-19 vaccination.

As keyworkers, Mummy and I can go for a weekly Covid-19 test to make sure that we are not unwittingly spreading the virus. I booked my vaccination appointment for 29th January. Mummy is not allowed the vaccine because she is pregnant.

**19th January 2021**
The deadliest day of the pandemic so far as 1,610 people lost their lives to Covid-19. What was that the media told us about being past the peak?

**20th January 2021**
A Wednesday, but Darcie was not able to go to Grandma and Grandad's. She had to self-isolate as a child she attends nursery with tested positive for Covid-19.

Yesterday's record for the number of deaths in a day was broken as 1,820 people died from coronavirus. Deaths are recorded as being caused by Covid-19 if someone dies within twenty-eight days of a positive test result. This can be slightly skewed if someone tests positive and is then hit by a bus less than four weeks later!

In international news, Joe Biden was sworn in as the 46th President of the United States of America, replacing Donald Trump.

**21st January 2021**
*I bless you'd on my hands!* you said after a snotty sneeze!

It is an amusing sight watching you feed Quartz before you go to nursery in a morning. *Be patient, Quartz!* you demanded as he climbed all over you, trying to get the pellets out of your hand!

**22nd January 2021**
You are starting to take more of an interest in the fact that Mummy is having a baby. You reckon that she is having twin girls! We hope not.

Each night, before you go to bed, you give Mummy a kiss before planting another one on her belly! Bless.

**23rd January 2021**
The weekend again. The limits on what we can actually do in a winter lockdown is becoming increasingly frustrating. During the first lockdown we were blindly grateful for the nice weather. And now here we are, locked down, in winter!

A Covid-19 television and radio advertisement has been released, challenging people to consider if they are doing everything they possibly can to prevent the spread of the virus. The impact of lockdown on people's mental health is possibly underestimated as to explicitly follow the rules would be enough to drive you insane!

**24th January 2021**
We are allowed to exercise outside once a day, with a maximum of one other person from another household. 'Social distancing' dictates that you must remain at least two metres apart from other people.

So, was you and I meeting Uncle Liam, Parry and Birchy at the park with five other children illegal? Lockdown restrictions do not apply to children under the age of fourteen years old, which you all were. The dads stayed at least two metres apart. Did that, therefore, make it legal?

Does that make sense? Confusing isn't it? We have lived in a state of confusion, alongside often contradictory guidelines, for the best part of a year. It still does not make any easier.

**26$^{th}$ January 2021**
On 11$^{th}$ November 2020, the UK recorded its 50,000$^{th}$ death from Covid-19. Today, just seventy-six days on, that total has doubled as more than 100,000 people have now been lost to the virus. Glaring evidence that coronavirus and its variants continue to have a devastating impact on people's lives.

**27$^{th}$ January 2021**
I was off work as Grandma and Grandad were supposed to go to Tenerife on holiday today. Theirs was one of the hundreds of thousands of holidays cancelled across the country as coronavirus continues to dampen any optimism.

You and I met Grandma, Grandad and Darcie at a country park. Spotting one another, you and Darcie ran towards each other from opposite ends of the path leading into the park. As you came together in a giggling embrace, Darcie exclaimed, *I have missed you, Noah!* It appeared to capture the isolation that people across the world are feeling as we live through these depressing times.

Boris Johnson announced that the Government will outline the 'roadmap' out of the current lockdown on 22$^{nd}$ February. There is a feeling that it will only be safe to reopen schools on 8$^{th}$ March, and not immediately after the February half-term as was first suggested. This is so that the most vulnerable people in society can achieve immunity from the virus through receiving their first dosage of the vaccine.

**28th January 2021**
Mummy and I went to the infirmary for the baby's first scan. We found out your baby brother or sister is due to be born on 8th August. When you got home from nursery we made a video of you holding the picture of the scan to send to people to share the news.

When Mummy asked, 'Who's having a baby?' you responded by saying, *Us!* This was followed by your forensic explanation of the scan picture. Pointing at the ultrasound, you exclaimed, *Look! There's the baby's back... and poo!*

**29th January 2021**
After work, I drove to the Greater Manchester Mass Vaccination Centre at the Etihad Campus for my first dose of the Oxford University/AstraZeneca vaccine.

The enormity of the pandemic hit me as I queued with hundreds of other people inside the Manchester Tennis and Football Centre. The clinical environment felt so surreal, and I became a small part of the largest vaccination rollout the country has ever seen.

More than 7.8 million people have now received their first dose of the vaccine in the United Kingdom.

**30th January 2021**
Feeling the side-effects of the vaccine – light-headedness and aching all over – was not helped by how loud and hyperactive you were all morning.

It was a bitterly cold day but we needed to go for a walk to collect some items for your nature topic at nursery.

The other day, given the lack of things to do, I intentionally failed to leave the cardboard bin out for collection so you and I could go and spend some father-son time at the tip!

### 2nd February 2021

In the very first few weeks of the pandemic, a ninety-nine-year-old World War Two veteran raised £32 million for the NHS by walking a hundred laps of his garden. Last July, he was knighted by Queen Elizabeth II at Windsor Castle.

Today, Captain Sir Tom Moore died of Covid-19, aged one hundred, in Bedford Hospital. It certainly signifies the dark times we are living through when the nation's shining light of the pandemic has now succumbed to the virus.

In brighter news, United became the first team in the Premier League to win 9–0 twice, beating Southampton at Old Trafford. I can remember United winning by the same scoreline twenty-six years ago against Ipswich Town, when Andy Cole scored five of the goals.

### 3rd February 2021

For weeks, Darcie has been telling everyone that she is having a baby. We thought that she had just been echoing our news but tonight Uncle Liam and Auntie Emma announced that they are due to have a baby in September.

At 6pm, we clapped on our doorstep with neighbours to remember Captain Sir Tom Moore.

The Government feel as though we are past the peak of the current wave of Covid-19 infections. The R rate is believed to have fallen to between 0.7 and 1.1. Ten million people have now received their first dosage of the vaccine.

**6th February 2021**
An absolutely awful day, weather-wise.

You and Mummy had a lie-in as I watched Joe Root become the first ever cricketer to score a double-hundred in their one hundredth Test match.

It has come to something when your daily exercise consists of running around B&Q, hiding in bathroom displays. Suppose you have to be creative when you are in lockdown.

We dropped a food parcel off for Great-Nana Mave on the way home, including some broccoli and cheddar soup you made with Mummy yesterday. Yes, that's right, broccoli and cheddar! Safe to say I swerved that particular dish!

The monotony of the cold, dark weekends is starting to take its toll and the end to this nightmare does not appear to be in sight. We do have to maintain a sense of perspective, though. As difficult as life can be at times we have not lost anyone close to us, which should not be underestimated.

**10th February 2021**
The Government has set a target of vaccinating fifteen million people by 15th February. This equates to one in four adults in the country. Two million vaccines have to be administered in the next five days for this target to be reached.

As of 15th February, all passengers arriving in the country from those on the Red List are requested to pay for, and self-isolate in, a hotel room at the airport for eleven nights. This will cost them £1,750.

The Red List is made up of the countries from which travel to the United Kingdom is banned. There are currently thirty-three countries on it. Moving forwards, countries could be added at very short notice. This represents the largest restriction on international travel that we have seen in our lifetime.

**12th February 2021**
Nationally, the R rate fell below 1 for the first time since last July. Is this a sign that the virus is slowing down? Or just representative of the fact that social contact has been severely reduced by the current lockdown? If that is the case, being locked down is working. But when will we be free again?

**15th February 2021**
Half-term so Mummy is off work all week and I am only working tomorrow. The fight against your boredom is proving to be a difficult one.

You are turning into something of a local legend at the tip. *See ya, lads!* you shouted to two blokes who worked there after you had helped empty cardboard out of my boot.

After lunch you helped to wash the cars. Your self-appointed job was to use the hosepipe to wash the bubbles away.

15.3 million people have now received their first Covid-19 vaccination. 230 people died today after testing positive for the virus, taking the total number of deaths to 117,396.

Ominously, we are being told by the Government that the journey out of this lockdown is going to be 'a cautious one'.

### 18th February 2021

*Four and a zero make forty!* you exclaimed from the back of my car, taking notice of the traffic signs.

'Well done, Noah! What does a 'two' and a 'zero' make?'

*Two-ty!*

Not quite, Little Man, but we understood your logic!

We went to Altrincham for lunch. We last went there on the weekend of your second birthday when we struggled to find a seat in the busy market hall. Fast forward fourteen months and the streets were deserted. The stalls selling hot food made it clear you had to move on once you had bought your lunch. We had to eat on the steps outside the market as all the benches had been taken away to preserve 'social distancing'.

You have a fantastic memory for a three-year-old. *I have been here before with Grandma and Grandad*, you proclaimed as we walked towards the entrance of Dunham Massey. You also remembered that when you last visited the lake was frozen over. We soon regretted not putting your waterproof all-in-one on when you fell forward into a muddy puddle!

In news away from coronavirus, NASA successfully landed the Perseverance Rover on the surface of Mars. The robot is designed to hunt for signs of past microbial life and is the first mission of its kind to the Red Planet since the 1970s.

The R rate is now reported to have dropped to between

0.6 and 0.9, the lowest it has been since May 2020. How will we keep this rate down when social restrictions are lifted? That is the question on everyone's lips.

## Chapter 17

# THE 'ROADMAP' TO NORMALITY

**22nd February 2021**

At nursery, the topics of the week were sharing, teamwork and being grateful. At story time, one of the nursery nurses read you and the rest of the children a book in which two dogs were competing at tennis.

*Dogs can't play tennis!* you declared, possibly remembering the human beings you saw contest the Australian Open Singles Finals at the weekend. After hearing your revelation, the class refused to be interested in the rest of the book!

At 7pm, Boris Johnson delivered the country's plan for moving out of lockdown. There are four steps to 'normality', each having to pass the following four tests before we can move on to the next:

The vaccine rollout continues to be successful.

The vaccine needs to reduce the number of deaths and people in hospital from Covid-19.

Infection rates must not risk a surge in hospitalisations, which would place additional pressure on the NHS.

New variants of the virus must not increase the risk of infection rates rising.

On 8th March all schools and colleges will see their pupils return. As part of the same stage, on 29th March, outdoor sports will be allowed to resume. We will also be able to meet in groups of up to six people, or with one other household, outdoors.

Step 2, which will kick in no earlier than 12th April, will see non-essential shops being allowed to open. This means that Grandma will be able to reopen her hairdressing salon. Restaurants, pubs and bars will also open for outdoor table service only.

Step 3, scheduled to start on 17th May, will mean that the 'rule of six', or two households, can be applied outdoors. Indoor hospitality will reopen and up to 10,000 people will be able to attend live sporting events.

The final step, if the previous three steps are successful, will come into force no earlier than 21st June. It is hoped that by this point, all legal limits on social contact will be removed. This will pave the way for people to attend large gatherings, such as football matches, pop concerts and weddings, as normal.

So, there's the plan. But as we have come to learn over the last twelve months, there is no guarantee that everything will go according to it. A spike in infections could result in us regressing so it needs to be approached with caution.

Let's hope that the light at the end of the proverbial tunnel is only four months away. Being optimistic about the prospect of freedom would have been incomprehensible this time last year. It is frightening how the mentality of the nation has been reconstructed in eleven months.

**24th February 2021**
Tiger Woods, widely regarded as the greatest golfer to have played the game, ended up in hospital after seriously breaking his leg in a car accident.

As I walked downstairs, you had pulled a chair up to the tropical fish tank. As you looked inside, you enquired, *Where are all my fishes?* Over a period of time, the fifteen or so fish in the tank had died and floated to the top. Hiding such loss from you was evidently a waste of energy as, unconcerned, you said, *Never mind. We will get some more.*

Grandma and Grandad had their Covid-19 jabs yesterday and ended up regretting not choosing a day that did not immediately precede looking after you and Darcie. Grandma claimed she could have cried when she saw that you had both emptied the card and board games over the playroom floor because you were *having a party!*

**25th February 2021**
I asked you why you were looking forward to coronavirus going away and you replied, *Diddikicks, beaches and... pubs!*

Shola Shoretire became United's youngest ever player to appear in European competition. He came on as a substitute, aged seventeen years and twenty-three days, in the Europa League against Real Sociedad. It is a shame Old Trafford was not full to witness it.

**27th February 2021**

It is clear that we need to be up and out at weekends as the same four walls at home transform you into a bored and restless state.

We met Grandma and Grandad at the park and bumped into Birchy, Matilda and Theo. We had never seen the park so busy! It kind of makes a mockery of not being able to have people in your back garden when you can go to a park with hundreds of other people! I understand the restrictions are there to stop people being wilfully ignorant but such experiences highlight the frustration of living through a third national lockdown.

**28th February 2021**

You have developed a dangerous fondness for jumping – up and down on your bed, from sofa to sofa and down the stairs. Mummy insisted that you promise not to continue when you landed a jump from the fifth step on the staircase down to the bottom! In truth, we were impressed rather than annoyed despite the risk involved!

For a change, it was a lovely sunny day and we went for a walk in the fields surrounding our house. The warmer weather cast our minds back to the relative enjoyment of the first lockdown. You were so happy to see your favourite horse, '*Tweaka*', again.

In the afternoon, you went for another walk with Stevie, Simon and Harley as Mummy and I went for an early gender scan in Trafford. We paid privately as we were unsure whether, due to restrictions in hospitals, I would be able to go with Mummy for the free ones!

Back at home, to reveal the news, we recorded a video

of you finding out that you were going to have a baby brother. As you pulled a baby-blue set of clothes out of a bag you were still adamant that you were having a little sister, something you had told everyone for weeks. You were clearly more interested in the *Paw Patrol* toy that your baby brother had 'bought' for you from Tesco.

So, in six months' time we will have a baby boy. All we need to work out now is his name!

**1st March 2021**
The pandemic has been shrouded in negativity, devastation and grief. Through all of that, the nation can be proud of the success of its vaccination programme. Over twenty million people have now received their first jab of the Covid-19 vaccine.

Your Great-Grandad Joe, who died in 2007, would have been eighty-six years old today.

**2nd March 2021**
Your problem-solving skills border on admirable. You now move the footstool, which you use to stand up and wee in the toilet, under the landing lights so you can turn them on and off.

Before bed, you brought the footstool down the stairs so you could open the fridge and pour your own cup of milk!

**3rd March 2021**
You and Darcie gatecrashed a television drama set under the bridge near the park. You were both fascinated by a blue car standing up with its bonnet stuck in the grass as well as a red car in the river.

You have become captivated by the woods at the back of Grandma and Grandad's house. *Foxes come out at the night time, Daddy, when we are in bed*, you told me.

Your Great-Grandad Charles 'Ronny', who passed away in 2000, would have celebrated his ninetieth birthday today.

### 4th March 2021

World Book Day. When Mummy dropped you off at nursery, it quickly became apparent to her that all the other children were in fancy dress! The guilt brought on from such forgetful parenting was short-lived as I delivered an emergency tiger onesie for you to get changed in to.

You were offered a place in the nursery class at our local primary school, starting in September. You are growing up too fast!

### 6th March 2021

*I have never been on a double-decker bus*, is what you have started to tell everyone. Such dreams are easily realised in lockdown, when weekends are not taken up by normal socialisation.

So, we drove into the town centre and boarded your first ever double-decker bus. On reflection, Mummy and I had not been on a bus in the town centre for perhaps more than half our lifetimes!

You were very excited and observant on the back of the top deck. Your preoccupation and anxiety built as you waited to press the 'Stop' button at the top of the road leading down to the country park where we were going. So much so, that you left your toy truck on board as we disembarked!

Given how distraught you were as we walked down to the park, Mummy started to work out how long it would take for the bus to reach its destination, turn round and come back. After a time-limited walk around the park we eventually missed the bus that had transported your toy fifteen miles through two towns and back. However, we managed to board the one following it.

Back in the town centre, I alighted our bus as quickly as I could and chased the toy-carrier half a mile up the road. The level of foresight, effort and determination was certainly lost on you as I delivered the mould of plastic and metal back to its rightful owner.

Walking back to the car, you told us, *I've never been on a tram*. Well, I suppose that's next weekend sorted!

Chapter 18

# 'ROADMAP': STAGE ONE

**8th March 2021 – 350 Days Since the Pandemic Began**
Millions of children and young people returned to school as part of the first phase of the Government's exit strategy from lockdown. There are different guidelines for different age groups. Some will have to wear face masks at all times and others will need to be tested for Covid-19 twice a week. Mummy has been taking twice-weekly Covid-19 tests at home since the start of the year.

In the evening, millions of people tuned into Oprah Winfrey's interview with Prince Harry and his wife, Meghan Markle. The couple are now living in the United States of America, having stepped back from their royal duties. The most sensational of their claims was that a member of the royal family expressed concern at how dark their baby son Archie's skin was going to be when he was born.

**9th March 2021**

The Olympic and Paralympic Games, scheduled to take place this summer in Tokyo, Japan, will go ahead with no overseas spectators due to coronavirus.

**11th March 2021**

The good news? Mummy won the Mother's Day raffle at nursery – a hamper – which was a double surprise because she did not know I had entered it on her behalf.

The bad news? You failed to keep your pants dry and had difficulty using your ears at nursery. We have been trying to address the latter for a while, counting loudly to three. Your apprehension as you feel the control slipping away as we approach 'three' often results in an emotional breakdown.

The solution? A chart where you can earn two stickers a day, one for staying dry and another for listening.

**13th March 2021**

*Look! It's white balling!*

'You mean hail stoning, Little Man?!'

Despite instructing me to cover your baked beans with mangetout at teatime, you proceeded to remove it all with one hand and take it off your plate! Not quite the *perfect meal* you had declared it to be beforehand, then?

**14th March 2021**

These crazy times have been with us for almost twelve months, and we are starting to come back round to days we remember so clearly from last year.

Today was Mother's Day. Last Mother's Day was the day before we were all told, for the first time, 'Stay at home'.

You bought Mummy, who you now refer to as *Pregosaurus*, a handheld vacuum cleaner and some tickets to see the comedian, Joel Dommett. Ironically, the second present was an excuse for me to spend some time alone with Mummy!

Just like the perfect son, you made Mummy a fruit salad for breakfast, haphazardly chopping melon, grapes and blueberries into a bowl.

We had a walk to the 'Gruffalo's Cave' and, as per usual, you collected items on the way. Today, it was a ram's horn which you carried the best part of three miles home!

Before bed, you had a go at being a doctor with your medical toy set. You took Mummy's temperature and, drawing the thermometer away from her ear, announced it had registered at *twenty past seven!* Priceless!

Mummy really enjoyed her last Mother's Day as the mother of one little boy. Next year, *Frog*, the name you have chosen for your little brother, will also be here!

### 15th March 2021

One hundred million Covid-19 tests have now been carried out in the United Kingdom.

It was a peaceful evening for Mummy and I as you fell asleep in the car on the way home from nursery. You woke up briefly at 9pm to put your pyjamas on and then drifted back off.

### 16th March 2021

There was no repeat of yesterday evening as you took forty-five minutes to work your way through the following bedtime routine. Having a bath, putting your pyjamas on, drying your hair, drinking a cup of milk, giving Quartz a kiss, reading Mummy a story, having me read you a story, stalling choosing a bedtime song, singing a bedtime song, brushing your teeth, giving me, Mummy and *Frog* a kiss and a *squeeze* and getting into bed.

Five minutes later, you appeared at the top of the stairs, and shouted, *Daddy! Can you tuck me in?*

### 20th March 2021

My thirty-fifth birthday. I'm now officially recognised as the first person in the family to have two birthdays affected by the Covid-19 pandemic.

We took you for a ride on your bike around the lake and you courteously roared, *Thank you!* to anyone who let you past.

You inevitably took a tumble after hurtling into the back of a couple. They subconsciously reached down to help you up before drawing sharply backwards, most certainly having remembered that such degrees of kindness are not 'Covid-secure'. How the world has changed in twelve months!

### 21st March 2021

We made the most of the slightly warmer weather and did some jobs outside in the garden. You were tasked with washing your filthy bike. This was going well until you got some soapy suds on your toy fire engine. It is astonishing to witness how something so inconsequential can lead to a devastating loss of emotion control!

The UK has now vaccinated more than half of its adult population and is on track to offer all adults at least one jab by the end of July.

**22nd March 2021**
You and I spent the day together as I was off work. By lunchtime, you had told me you loved me three times. You are such a loving little boy.

We went for a walk around the reservoir and had a picnic. As you sat on a bench tucking into your feast, a couple of rotund women walked past us. Your thoughts engaged your mouth and you opined, *Maybe their babies are in their tummy.*

Today, seventeen people died of Covid-19. This was the lowest daily figure since 28th September 2020. Encouraging news, even as we acknowledge that lockdown remains entirely justified.

**23rd March 2021 – A Year Since Lockdown Began**
Today marked exactly a year since Boris Johnson made his famous speech on television, ordering everyone to 'Stay at home'. Since then, we have endured two further lockdowns and suffered restrictions and regulations which have impacted all areas of daily life.

A total of 149,117 people in the UK have sadly had coronavirus disease recorded on their death certificate.

At 12 noon, people from all corners of the country stopped what they were doing to hold a minute's silence to remember those that have succumbed to the virus. At 8pm, people stood on their doorsteps with mobile phones, torches and candles to signify a 'beacon of remembrance'.

As we move forward, there are concerns that a third wave of Covid-19 may be on the horizon. The vaccination supplies have been curtailed due to falling production rates in India. In France, Germany and Italy, positive cases of Covid-19 are on the rise.

No one is any clearer about whether they will be able to enjoy unrestricted family holidays abroad this summer. Even so, a sense of perspective is required.

## 24th March 2021

*Why is it morning time so quick?* you asked sleepily as Mummy woke you up for nursery.

From today, the 'stay at home' advice has been relaxed. We are now being told to 'stay local'. Outdoor sports can resume and we are allowed to socialise with up to six people, or two households, outside.

In the last twenty-four hours, twenty-three people have died of Covid-19. There were also 4,654 positive recorded cases.

The vaccination programme has now delivered thirty million first doses to people across the country.

Yesterday morning, the clocks went forward an hour. This means that it now stays lighter for longer at bedtime. Trying to explain that you will be going to bed in the light for the next six months was difficult as you protested, *It is not night-time!*

## 30th March 2021

You are becoming very fond of bugs. When I picked you up from nursery you told me all about the *baby ladybird* you had found *with a sore wing*.

Mummy was late home from work. With it being a nice evening, we enjoyed a chippy tea in the back garden. You were not for letting me sit down at the table because it meant destroying a spider's web! You need signing up for the Royal Entomological Society!

**1st April 2021**
A study has revealed that, despite living through a pandemic for more than a year, only 52% of people can correctly identify the main symptoms of Covid-19.

Just in case your Mummy reads this, I suppose I must reference that it was our fifth wedding anniversary today!

**6th April 2021**
A bitterly cold day. Yesterday morning, there was actually snow on the ground.

You have had a cough for the last few days so we had to pin you down on the sofa to do a Covid-19 test. For you, this means a plastic swab being inserted up your nose, as opposed to adults having to swab both nostrils as well as the back of their throats. Still, it was an experience that led to lots of arm-thrashing and squirming from you. Once we had taken the sample we needed you screamed, *I don't like Mummy and Daddy anymore!*

The test was negative but, coincidentally, I had to take you to the doctor's for your routine set of vaccinations. It transpired that Mummy had sent us a day and five minutes early, causing you an element of confusion.

*Daddy... why have I not had my jabs?* you enquired, as we trudged back to the car. This was followed by *Silly Mummy!* through the hands-free in the car after we informed her of her mistake.

After such a medically-themed morning we went to Bolton Abbey in Skipton for a 'Bunny Hunt'. Crossing the stepping stones over the River Wharfe seemed a good idea until we reached the halfway point. There, a few of the stones were not level and spaced a bit too far apart. The water was deep and the air was too cold for it to be funny to fall in!

After some balancing and careful problem-solving, against your cries of *I don't want to go in the water* and *I want to use the bridge!* the three of us made it safely to the opposite riverbank. Eating a well-deserved snack on the other side, we watched some other people who were not so lucky!

### 9<sup>th</sup> April 2021
Prince Philip, Duke of Edinburgh, reigning Queen Elizabeth II's husband and consort of seventy-three years, died at home in Windsor Castle. He was ninety-nine years old.

It is becoming a habit for you to make the front room as dark as possible, turning the lights off and closing the curtains, when you are watching television. Someone is going to enjoy going to the cinema!

In the garden, you shouted in surprise whilst pointing upwards, *Look! An aeroplane!* Jet fuel trails have gone from being such a common feature of the skies above our heads to rarities throughout the pandemic.

You then told us that you do not want to go on holiday anymore due to coronavirus. We decided not to press you for an explanation in the hope that such feeling would naturally dissipate when the time comes to use air travel as a family once again.

### 10<sup>th</sup> April 2021
Once the initial excitement of having a baby brother

settled down, Mummy and I decided not to talk about him too much so that you could develop your own affection for your little brother. It has certainly worked! You now talk about him more than we do, kissing Mummy's tummy and talking about how he is *eating Mummy's food to grow*.

In typical cheeky fashion, you have now started to blame your baby brother when you burp or break wind!

In the afternoon, we went to Darcie's house to watch the Grand National. Uncle Liam and I backed the winning horse, Minella Times, as Rachael Blackmore became the first female jockey to win the famous race.

**11$^{th}$ April 2021**
Overnight, a thick covering of snow had fallen. This provided you with even more encouragement to be mischievous. Driving to B&Q, you pelted a snowball at me using snow that had fallen inside the car! Walking across the car park, I had to prevent you from throwing snowballs at strangers, cars and into the store!

Chapter 19

## 'ROADMAP': STAGE TWO

**12th April 2021**
As of today, non-essential shops can open. Grandma Buckley opened her hairdressing salon for the first time in months.

Indoor sport can now resume which means you will be back at Diddikicks on Sunday. Pubs, bars and restaurants can now serve food and drink – outdoors only – but people must only socialise in a groups of six or as two households together.

When I got home from work you told me, *I have banged my head three times!* Two of these occasions you had made up but your bump from jumping into the frame of Great-Nana Mave's armchair, excited for your chippy tea, was clearly visible!

**15th April 2021**
Nana Roz looked after you last night so Mummy and I could enjoy a spa night at a hotel. After she dropped you

off we drove to Waddington and enjoyed a meal out for the first time since we were in Whitby, almost six months ago! On reflection, eating out is a luxury. However, having to wait so long highlights the unpredictability of what lies ahead in a pandemic.

We chose The Waddington Arms for lunch because it has a slide and a climbing frame in the beer garden. A slide you were pulled from on several occasions for not listening to our instructions to not go down on your front!

You were playing nicely with a little girl and proudly told her, *My Daddy drives a Volkswagen Golf!* Not a bad effort for your first ever chat-up line!

### 16th April 2021

Your presence with Grandad Col and I at the driving range, complete with your little 7-iron and red-and-white plastic golf balls, raised a few smiles from people. Your awareness of what is going on around you is certainly not at a level where just one adult can supervise you in an environment where people are swinging clubs and hitting balls! You kept wanting to run onto the range to chase the golf balls!

Mummy took you to the dentist and you were told you had *sparkly teeth* and received every little boy and girl's dream – a sticker! All the hours spent drilling a routine into you in the bathroom are paying off!

### 18th April 2021

Diddikicks returned. Fortunately, there was no roleplaying of witches or Father Christmas from the coaches, games which have created such fear and upset for you in the past.

Mummy went for a walk and some lunch with friends so you spent the afternoon playing sport with me in the garden – football, tennis, cricket and rugby.

Back on 15th November, me and a group of my mates from around the country and other parts of the world, *the lads* as you call them, started a beer tournament over video conference. This began with thirty-two branded beers and had become a regular feature of Sunday afternoons ever since. Each week, a group of us have sat and chatted at our computer screens, often watching live football at the same time, drinking two ties. Today was the final and, as you have done for the past five months, you sat on my knee for parts of the conversation. For the record, Heineken beat Krombacher 6–4 to be crowned the champion beer.

Today, as United beat Burnley 3–1, news broke that twelve clubs from across the continent, United included, were breaking away to form a European Super League that would rival the current UEFA Champions League. The anger this evoked from within the football community was phenomenal.

### 20th April 2021

Your manager at nursery is fasting for the Islamic holy month of Ramadan. Exploring this with you, you told Mummy that fasting is *when you eat at night*.

I had my second Covid-19 jab at the Greater Manchester vaccination centre.

Uncle Liam and Auntie Emma found out that they are having a baby boy. Whilst Darcie was elated, you were less happy. You said that your cousin, due less than a month after your own baby brother, will be *stinky*. Finally, after much persuasion, you brought yourself round to saying *'latulations* (congratulations) to your auntie and uncle in a video message!

**21$^{st}$ April 2021**
On 25$^{th}$ May last year, a black American man named George Floyd died after a white police officer knelt on his neck whilst arresting him. George's death sparked a worldwide publicisation of the Black Lives Matter movement. Before every Premier League match since, the vast majority of players have taken a knee and raised a fist in support of the movement. Today, we woke to the news that the police officer had been found guilty of George's murder in Minneapolis, United States of America.

Referring to yourself as a *cool dude*, Daddy dropped you off at Grandma and Grandad's in a cap and sunglasses. Off you went to Lytham St Anne's and Bispham for the day. Now the weather is getting better, there is so much more you and Darcie can do with your grandparents on a Wednesday.

Grandma had to wash your white trainers when you got back because you got stuck in *sinking sand* on the beach.

After the outrage that followed the announcement of a potential European Super League, all six English clubs – Arsenal, Chelsea, Liverpool, Manchester City, Manchester United and Tottenham Hotspur – withdrew from the plans. By the end of the day, only three of the twelve clubs that signed up to the idea remained.

**22$^{nd}$ April 2021**
Over one in five adults in the country have now received their second dose of the Covid-19 vaccination.

Not that we told you this, but we nearly lost Quartz today. He was playing in the garden and escaped through a small gap at the side of the garage. Luckily, I found him in a neighbouring garden and chased him back to where he belongs!

## 23rd April 2021

When you go to the park and ride your bike you refuse to take your helmet off when playing in the play area. Perhaps not such a bad idea when considering how accident-prone you are. With Nana Roz today, you tried to ride your bike up the slide!

I achieved a promotion at work – or a *potion* as you called it – so we went to Grandma and Grandad's with Uncle Liam, Auntie Emma and Darcie to celebrate.

## 24th April 2021

Swimming started back up again. It is a mystery why Covid-19 prevents Mummy from being able to get in the pool with you, or enter the building at all, when you are allowed one adult with you at Diddikicks. Mummy has to drop you off at the fire exit ready to swim and collect you from the same point when you have finished.

In the afternoon, we went for a walk on the moors to see the windmills. You correctly counted twenty-three of them on the way up to the top. You were more proud, however, of the fact that you managed to fall over ten times on the way back down. *I'm clumsy!* was your honest admission.

## 25th April 2021

Grandma took you to Diddikicks so that Mummy and I could help Grandad wallpaper your bedroom.

The sticky crab, won at the arcade on the pier at Saltburn-by-the-Sea back in October, has lived on the dashboard of my car ever since. The warmer weather has now turned it into a gooey mess. I brought it into the house where you spent half an hour throwing it against every surface you could see before laying it to rest in the bin.

Whilst the number of Covid-19 cases are falling in our country, the same cannot be said for other nations around the world. India recorded 346,786 cases today, with 2,624 deaths. This was the highest daily death total anywhere in the world since the pandemic began.

## 27th April 2021 - 400 Days Since Lockdown Began

Toddler life can switch from laughs and giggles to total turmoil in an instant. Life was wonderful from the moment you woke up but when the time came to leave the house for nursery you were screaming about how you are not friends with Mummy and Daddy anymore! Only the shock of your seatbelt bursting open as I drove off our estate stopped you from crying.

You can be kind and considerate as well, choosing Mummy's favourite book, *Monkey Puzzle*, for her to read to you at bedtime.

## 29th April 2021

Anything that has happened in the past, you refer to as occurring *yesterday*. At nursery, you vividly recalled the story of the first time you went on a double-decker bus to one of the nursery nurses. So impressed by your level of detail, she thought that it had actually happened yesterday!

**30th April 2021**
Pointing at the wrinkles on Mummy's forehead, you asked, *What are those?* This was followed up by enquiring, *Why have you got a hole?* as you pointed to a spot of the side of her head. Just say it as you see it, Little Man!

This week, it was Mummy's turn to get a promotion. I picked you up from Nana Roz's and we called in Tesco to buy Mummy some flowers. As we discussed what to buy Mummy, two ladies laughed out loud when you suggested, *Let's buy Mummy a dress!*

Yesterday, the carpet was laid in your 'big boy' bedroom. Despite your bed still needing to be delivered, you insisted on moving straight in and sleeping on your mattress on the floor. It was your first night in your new bedroom.

**2nd May 2021**
There were only six other children at Diddikicks. Possibly a sign that people were starting to get away again for the bank holiday weekend. On your way into the sports hall, a man asked you who your favourite player is. *Daddy*, was your simple, one-word response.

In the afternoon, we went to the golf club for a BBQ. Of all the things you could have chosen to eat you went for a sausage muffin with ketchup on.

At one point, you moved yourself under the table to play with your cars, not wanting to share with Daddy's friend Jordan's six-month-old son Jenson who had taken an interest in them!

United's game against Liverpool at Old Trafford was postponed because of fan protests against the Glazer family's ownership of the club, as well as United's original plans to form part of the European Super League. In wholly unsavoury scenes, several hundred fans broke into the stadium and protested on the pitch. This led to the match being called off by the police in the interests of player safety.

### 3rd May 2021

The horrendous weather gave us little choice but to go to IKEA – *No, Daddy… it's 'Eye-kea!'* – to buy some furniture for your bedroom. We tried and failed to find somewhere to eat lunch under shelter from the rain so we ended up taking a chippy home.

The Snooker World Championship Final became the first sporting event in the country to have a capacity crowd since the Cheltenham Horse Racing Festival in March last year. Mark Selby beat Shaun Murphy 18–5 to win his fourth world championship title.

### 4th May 2021

In the coming weeks the Government will release the Green List of countries to which holidaymakers can travel without having to quarantine on their return. However, a poll has found out that only 13% of people actually want to go abroad this year.

You are having to be discouraged from weeing in the bathroom jug after you have had a shower. Daddy asked why you then poured it down the sink, and not the bath, to which you answered bluntly, *'Cos there's toys down there!*

Just throw your urine into the place we all wash our faces then, Little Man!

### 5th May 2021

On the drive to drop you off at Grandma and Grandad's, I asked what animals you were looking forward to seeing at the zoo. *Tigers... and ants!* was your peculiar response.

Grandma took you to Chester Zoo with her friend Carol and Darcie. You were disappointed that the lions and tigers were asleep but you enjoyed seeing a panther and some bears, particularly the baby one.

It is a joy to watch the evolving relationship you have with your cousin Darcie, laughing, crying, playing and fighting with each other. You are also very adept at winding one another up.

*My brother is going to be called Ralphie*, Darcie announced on the journey home.

Your response of, *No he's not. My brother is going to be called Ralphie!* led to an extended period of bickering in the back of Grandma's car.

### 6th May 2021

*Daddy? Are you coming to wake me up?!* you shouted from your bed.

I was not around, because I had left the house at 6am to work in a polling station for the Local Council and Regional Mayoral Elections.

After nursery you and Mummy went to Great-Nana Mave's for a chippy tea as I was at a primary school nearby. As you walked round to drop some food off for me you told Mummy, *Ooooh! It is picking up.*

'What is?' Mummy asked.

*The wind!*

We do not know where you get some of your phrases from, this one making you sound sixty years older than you actually are!

## 7th May 2021

You stumbled into our bedroom at 5.55am moaning, *You did not put my pyjamas on!* No? That is what happens when you fall asleep in the car home and do not wake up, Little Man! You were swiftly sent back to bed.

Your confusion over the time of day continued when, forty-five minutes later, you returned whining, *But you've not read me a bedtime story!* So, to appease you, I read you a morning story instead.

As Nana Roz gave you your breakfast, she informed you that you were not going to see Great-Nana Mave today. *Why?* you asked. *'Cos of coronavirus?* A pandemic can consume the thoughts of the youngest of minds.

After polishing off your Cheerios, fruit and yoghurt you were given a baby wipe for your face. Cleaning yourself up you remarked, *Hands. Face. Space*, which is one of the slogans banded about to try and reduce the spread of Covid-19.

After being in lockdown for more than a quarter of your life, the virus and the language and terminology associated with it is becoming a normal part of your everyday speech.

## 8th May 2021

An absolutely horrendous day of torrential rain. So, there was not much to do other than go shopping.

When we bought some new fish a few weeks ago, you

wanted an Olaf ornament, from the Disney film *Frozen*, to go in your tank. Olaf is now starting to turn green with algae so we bought a catfish to clean the inside of the tank.

After declaring your excitement at the possibility of seeing ants at Chester Zoo, we bought you an ant farm. Life in a pandemic is evidently broadening mine and Mummy's minds about what to waste our money on! We ordered the ants online and they will arrive in the post next week.

### 9th May 2021

I got up in the early hours of the morning to watch Saúl 'Canelo' Álvarez fight Billie Joe Saunders for the WBO super middleweight title. It took place at the AT&T Stadium in Arlington, Texas, the home of the Dallas Cowboys American football team, in front of a US record crowd of 73,126. Signs, maybe, that the world is slowly moving back to normal. It does make one wonder why such crowds cannot safely attend sporting events over here though.

You did well at Diddikicks, dribbling – *little kicks* – faster and starting to change direction with the ball. You still worked yourself up over one of the games, becoming panicked and upset because Coach Zain was pretending to be a 'Hungry Hippo' and eating footballs.

I watched United at a drinking establishment for the first time this calendar year, under a gazebo in the car park outside the wine bar. They beat Aston Villa 3-1, with goals from Bruno Fernandes, Mason Greenwood and Edinson Cavani.

**10th May 2021**

You were in a very giddy mood when I picked you up from nursery. My friend Sucky, whose house we are going to be staying at in Scotland in June, called round to see us. You played up, acting daft and taking about *poo* and *widgies*.

You have got a new book, to help you understand Mummy's pregnancy, called *There's A House Inside My Mummy*. She read this to you at bedtime and you talked to your baby brother through Mummy's *tummy telephone*.

**12th May 2021**

Your Queen Ant, and her brood, arrived in the post yesterday so she is now settling into your ant farm.

You went to the park with Grandma and Grandad. You and Darcie came home filthy, which is always the sign of a good day.

At home, you asked me, *Daddy, we're mates aren't we?*

'Of course we are, Little Man. Who else is your mate?'

*Grandad Col. 'Cos he's a boy!*

A brief, explorative conversation revealed you think you can only be mates with boys. Your Mummy has her fingers crossed it stays the same for some time yet!

**13th May 2021**

Darcie's third birthday. She is now the only person in our family who has celebrated more birthdays in lockdown than she has outside of a pandemic.

As we encouraged you to write Darcie's birthday card, we tried to get you to think of some nice things to say about your cousin. We certainly did not write *she doesn't share*, which is what you kept suggesting!

We went to Darcie's house for tea where you enjoyed

playing with her new presents. You got spoilt for dessert, getting a portion of Darcie's vegan option, as she is allergic to dairy products, as well as your own.

Your compliments towards Darcie continued on the way home, calling her a *meanie* because she would not give you a kiss and a hug goodbye.

**14th May 2021**
You went shopping with Nana Roz and Great-Nana Mave and then to Mummy's 'Auntie' Shelley's house. Anthony, who Mummy grew up with, was visiting for the day with his children. Despite having never met them, your sociable nature meant you played really nicely.

With the country set to move into the 'roadmap's' third stage out of lockdown in three days, the Indian variant of Covid-19 is causing concern. If this proves to be more transmissible than the Kent strain, currently the most dominant in the United Kingdom, then it could halt our plans to slowly move out of lockdown.

**15th May 2021**
Mummy and I went out on our own for the first time since last September. It is inconceivable, having never lived through a pandemic before, that we would be forced to go so long without enjoying a meal and a few drinks together. Our choice of activity would also not have been sitting outside, under a shelter in the pouring rain.

The FA Cup Final was played at Wembley Stadium in front of a crowd of 20,000 – the biggest attendance at a sporting event in the United Kingdom since March 2020. Leicester City beat Chelsea 1–0.

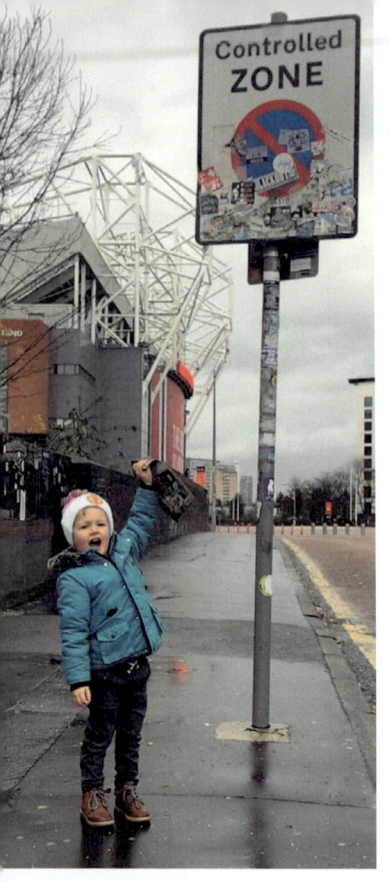

*'United We Stand! Out today!' Auditioning to be a fanzine seller on your first ever walk down Sir Matt Busby Way to Old Trafford.*

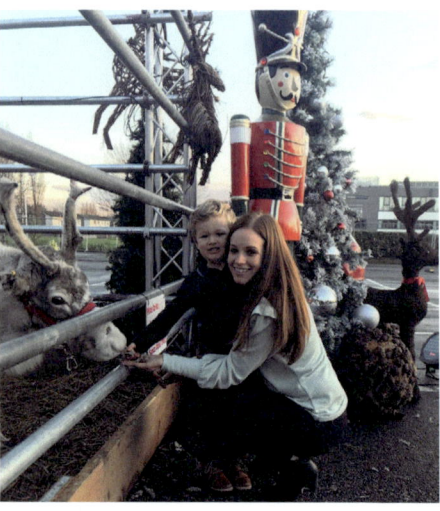

*Lockdown brought out so much innovation, imagination and creativity. This drive-thru 'Santa's Grotto', where we went on your third birthday, failed on all three counts!*

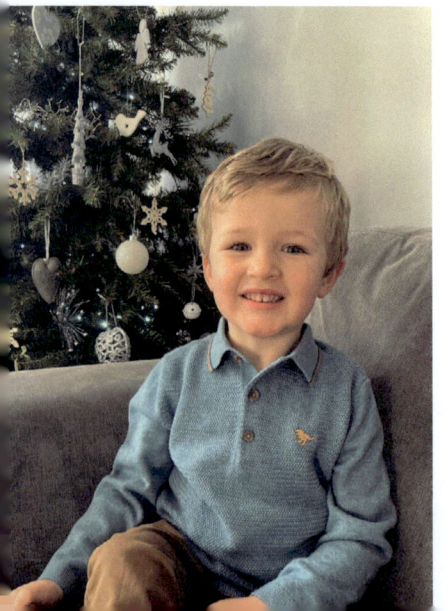

*Christmas Day 2020. We watched you grow up so much in the first nine months of lockdown.*

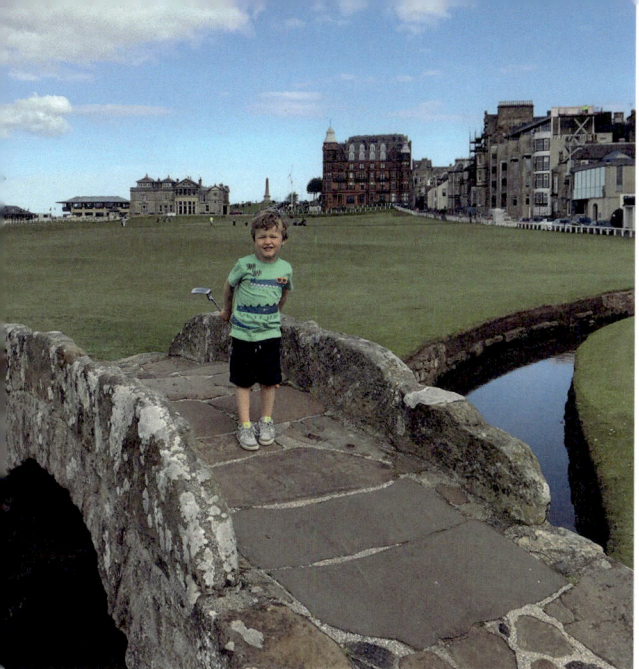

*On the Swilcan Bridge that crosses the 1st and 18th holes on The Old Course, St. Andrew's. You were desperate to try out your new putter.*

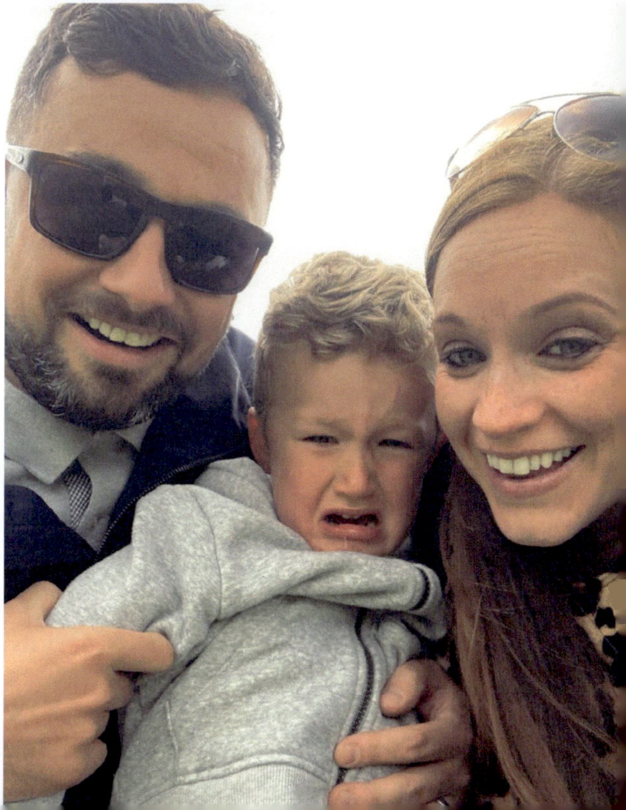

*Devastation after realising a bet does not always equal a winning horse.*

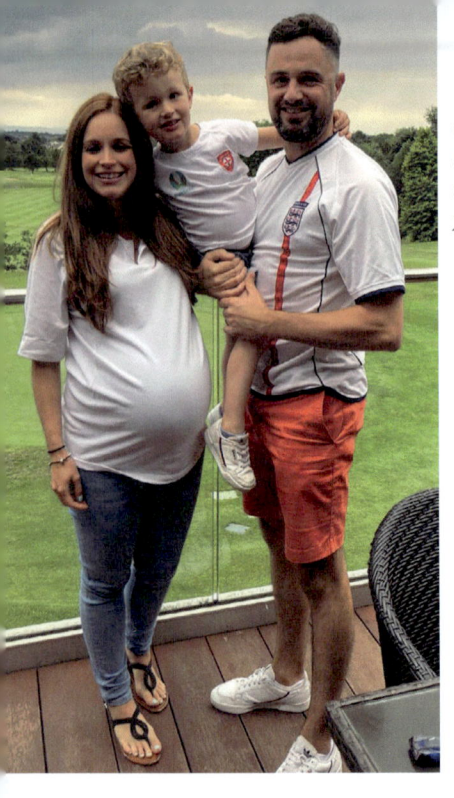

*On the balcony at the golf club before the Euro 2020 Final. It was not England's night, something you remembered for many weeks.*

*This was the first, but not the last, time you jammed your knee in the headboard of your new bed!*

*Adopting Thai pleasantries on the way out of the restaurant. This was the last picture I took of you as an only child.*

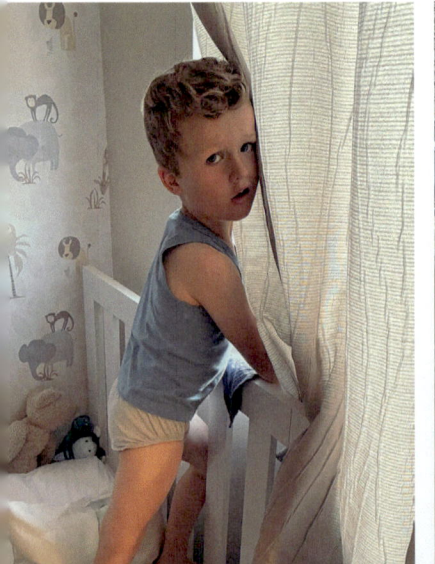
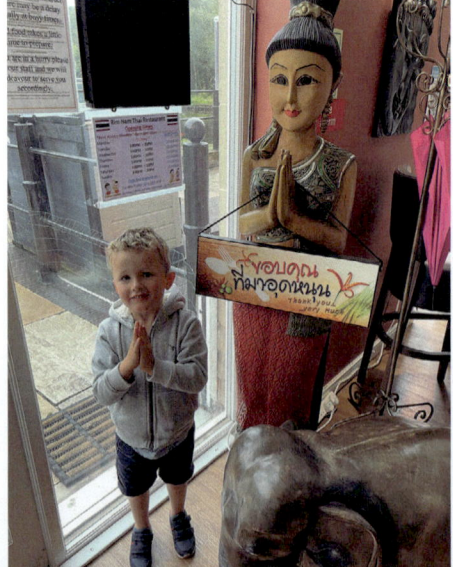

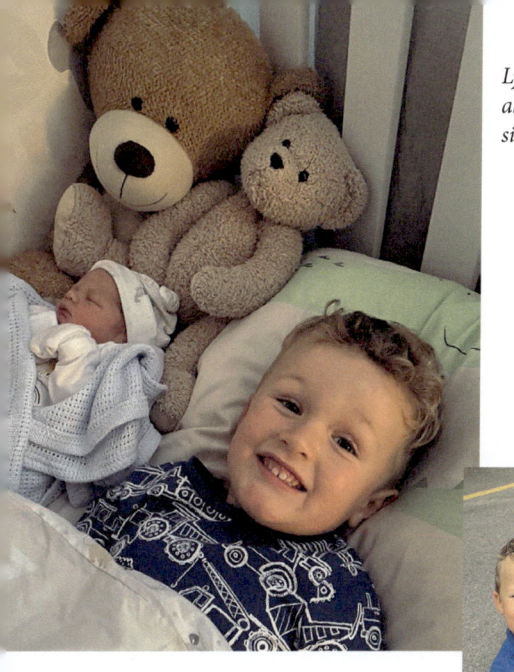

*Lying proudly in your bed alongside Xander Joseph, aged sixteen hours.*

*Pushing Xander in his pram on the way to your first day at school nursery.*

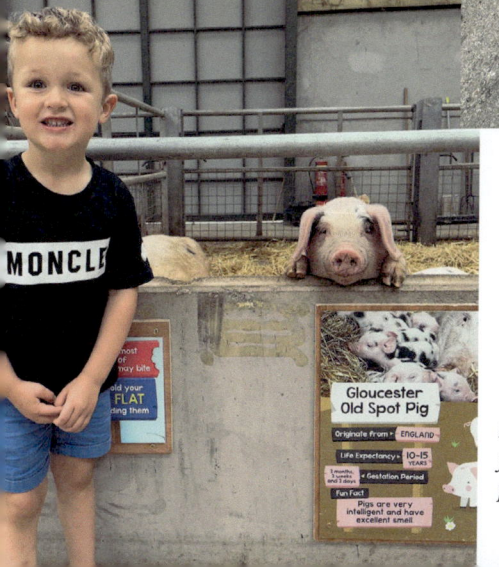

*Photobombed by a pig at the farm. One of my favourite pictures of the pandemic.*

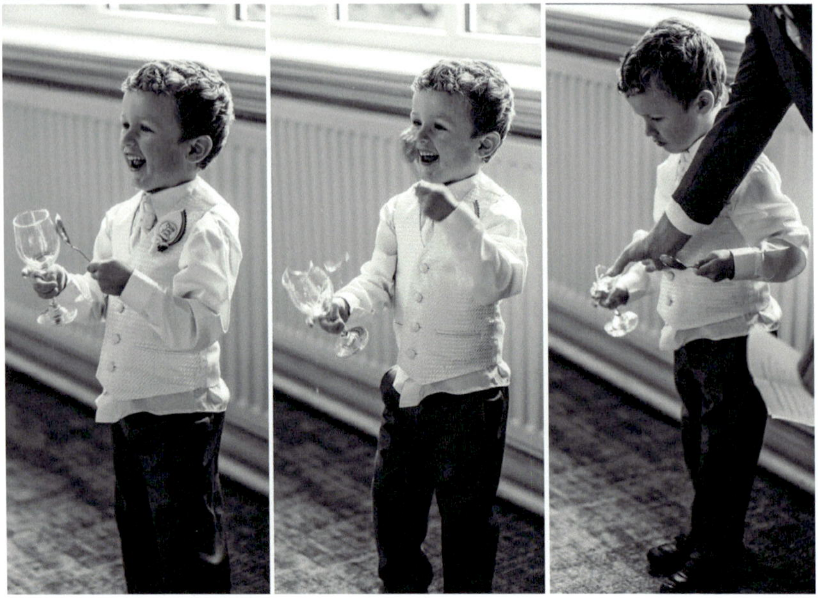

*Your attempt at imitating my glass-clinking as the Master of Ceremonies at Nana Roz and Nana James' wedding ended with shards of glass on the floor.*

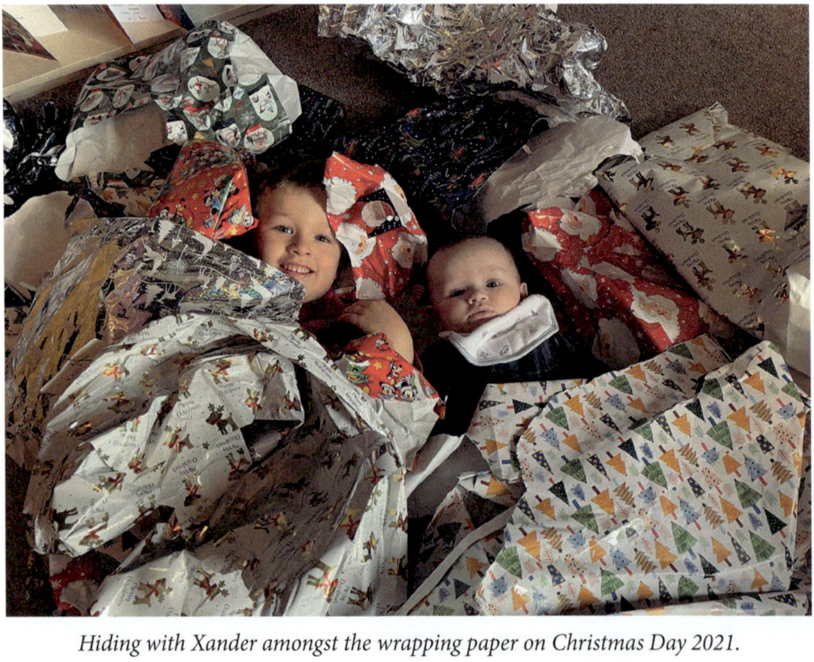

*Hiding with Xander amongst the wrapping paper on Christmas Day 2021.*

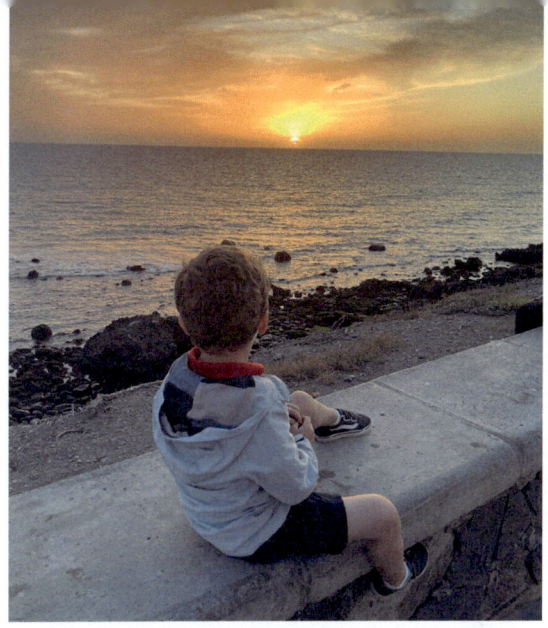

*Gazing as the sun sets into the Atlantic Ocean from Meloneras, Gran Canaria. We would return from this holiday to a new home for you to spend the rest of your childhood.*

*Xander was not the final addition to our family. Luca Jude Buckley was welcomed into our lives on 12th April 2024.*

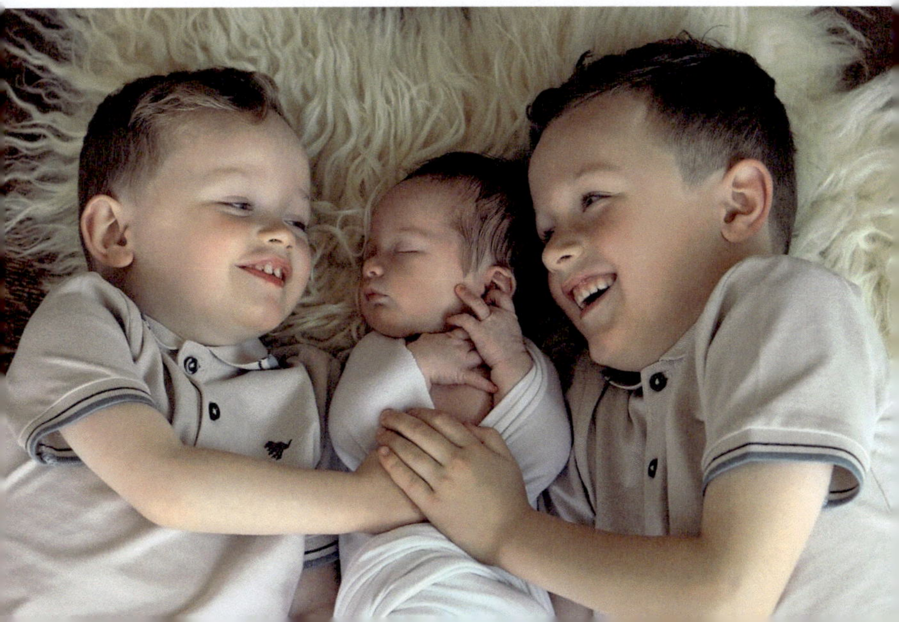

*Chapter 20*

# 'ROADMAP': STAGE THREE

**17th May 2021**
People are now allowed to socialise indoors, in homes, restaurants, pubs and cafés, in groups of six. Groups of up to thirty people are allowed to socialise outside. There is a general feeling that we are nearing the end of lockdown restrictions. The scheduled date for the end of all limits on social contact is Monday 21st June. However, the Indian variant of the virus looms large over any plans to enjoy absolute freedom once again.

People are now able to travel abroad, without quarantining on their return, to countries on the Green List.

Ironically, as social contact rules ease Mummy, due to being pregnant, is no longer teaching her class in school because it is more difficult for younger children to socially distance.

Today, you moaned to Mummy that you *want a job*. So

now, your job is to set the table each evening before we sit down for our tea.

### 18th May 2021

Last weekend you released the butterflies that arrived at our house a few weeks ago as a tub of caterpillars. You were very gentle holding them, placing them on the flowers so they could fly away. You even gave one a kiss!

Our conversation on the way to nursery was consumed by a discussion around what could have made a hole in the leaf you found on the drive. This took you back to the caterpillars and memories of the butterflies we released into the wild. With a sad frown you told me, *I miss my butterflies. They were my pets!*

Fans were able to attend a match at Old Trafford for the first time since 8th March 2020. They were treated to a forty-yard strike from Edinson Cavani as United only managed a 1–1 draw with Fulham.

The following morning, sensing you would be impressed by the goal, I showed it you on the television. It had the reverse effect as you moaned, *But I cannot kick it that far!*

### 20th May 2021

*Daddy! Darcie tried to put her tongue in her 'fostril'!* meaning one of the external openings of her nose, you exclaimed whilst sat on the toilet.

You have now started to make your bed in a morning. Which actually is not too difficult considering that it is still a mattress on the floor.

As you did two days ago, you fell asleep in the car on

the way home from nursery. It is amazing that we can transfer you into bed and you sleep until the following morning! Mummy and I then enjoyed some strange, early evening peace whilst you recuperated from an active day at nursery.

### 21st May 2021

Mummy was running late to pick you up from Nana Roz and James'. Nana Roz jokingly suggested it was because she had gone to the pub. *No. My Mummy doesn't go to the pub. My Daddy goes to the pub!*

I went to Darcie's house after work to drop some things off for her garden party tomorrow. Darcie was very excited and, as I was leaving, she kindly said, *You can come to my party, Uncle Aaron. But make sure you bring Noah!*

Mummy brought home some two-day-old chicks from work which you absolutely loved. *They are so cute!* you kept repeating as you sat holding them on your knee.

Mummy's tummy has grown to the point that you can no longer sit on her knee as comfortably as the chicks can on yours!

### 22nd May 2021

Uncle Liam and Auntie Emma decided to take advantage of the further relaxation of lockdown restrictions by hosting a belated garden party for Darcie's birthday. There was a bouncy castle outside which some of the adults enjoyed more than the children! It felt oddly liberating being able to socialise in a larger group with family and friends, some of whom we had not seen for a long time. Does this mean we are edging towards normality? Maybe.

### 23rd May 2021

The social impact of Covid-19, on even the youngest in society, was sadly apparent at Diddikicks. You and another little boy went to give one another a 'high five' and, in a strange moment of hesitation, glanced over to your daddies as if seeking approval to touch one another's hands. Proof, perhaps, that the pandemic has pervaded almost every conscious individual on the planet.

It is Grandad Col's birthday tomorrow so we went to a restaurant for tea. The socially distant tables, as well as having to wear face masks when not sat down at your table, means that eating out is still not quite the same.

It was raining, but that did not stop you and Darcie playing outside on the green. We knew that it was time go when Darcie fell off a small wall.

United beat Wolves 2–1 at Molineux to become only the fourth top-flight team to go an entire league season unbeaten away from home.

In other sporting news, Phil Mickelson, aged fifty, became the oldest golfer in history to win a major championship, winning the USPGA Championship by two shots at Kiawah Island, South Carolina.

### 24th May 2021

Grandad Col's sixty-first birthday.

We discovered that Darcie's tumble off the wall yesterday resulted in a broken arm! After nursery she came to see the chicks with a cast on. She called her injury a *'fwacture'*!

**25th May 2021**
Your nursery celebrated its twenty-fifth birthday so you went dressed smartly in a shirt and jeans for a party. Nursery's mascot is Zen the Zebra, which caused you to be confused about how a teddy can be twenty-five years old!

After being told that headbutting is not appropriate under any circumstances, you have developed your own special move, the *belly butt*, which involves you charging at me with your belly button leading the way!

**26th May 2021**
You were left at Grandma and Grandad's with the message 'Be gentle with Darcie' firmly instilled. *Why?* is your general response to any instruction these days

United lost the Europa League Final to Villarreal 11–10 on penalties following a 1–1 draw after extra-time. The less said about the whole debacle, the better.

**27th May 2021**
I picked you up from nursery just after lunch and took you to the indoor minigolf. On one hole you somehow managed to lose a ball by hitting it the wrong way through a revolving wheel. Walking back through the town centre, you kept loudly repeating, *I winned at golf*, much to the amusement of people passing by.

At the car park, you picked up a white dandelion and gave it a kiss. I turned round to see your contorted, spluttering face not enjoying the taste or texture of the seeds!

**28th May 2021**
You love a bit of gardening, or just getting your hands dirty in general, so at Great-Nana Mave's you helped her plant some sunflowers.

You also like to go about things in an unconventional manner. At the park with Nana Roz you thought it was a good idea to walk up the slide. This led to you slipping and landing on your face! Looking after you often feels like a challenge to keep you alive!

**29th May 2021**
Mummy brought you to pick me up from the golf club and you were in a very grumpy mood. You eventually came upstairs but not even the sight of Grandad Col walking up the eighteenth fairway cheered you up. Once you had settled down you took a great interest in the prize boards. I took a picture of you next to Great-Grandad Alan's name from when he won a Board Prize in the early 1990s.

Mummy went out with her friends so you had a night in with me and *the lads* for the Champions League Final. Chelsea beat Manchester City 1–0 to win European football's elite prize for the second time.

Boris Johnson, the country's prime minister throughout the whole of this pandemic, got married to Carrie Symonds. Due to the Covid-19 restrictions, there were only thirty guests at their wedding.

**31st May 2021**
Knowing we were going on holiday, you walked into Mummy and Daddy's bedroom first thing in the morning and asked, *Please can we go to the beach now?*

Our plan was not to go to the beach but, considering you also requested that we get on an *airport bus*, we decided to stop at a beach en route to the north east of England to soften the blow of not getting on a plane.

Every stone that you picked up on the pebbly shoreline in Seaham was, to your mind, *interesting*. You fancied yourself as a bit of a rock climber, forgetting that Mummy was seven months pregnant, clambering over the rough terrain and asking her to follow.

Further up the road in Durham, the weather was baking hot. It was hard work trying to find somewhere to stop and have a drink outside, given that in such times everyone has the same idea. Avoiding having to queue with a three-and-half-year-old, we found some seats outside the back of a hotel on the river.

Walking through the underground car park to start the next leg of our journey, you loved how your voice echoed off the low ceilings. Your shouts of *Hello! Hello!* were interrupted by a loud burp which you politely followed up with *Pardon me!* Where on Earth did we get you from?!

Once we got to our hotel for the night in Newcastle-upon-Tyne you excitedly searched for our room, scoured the room's facilities and claimed the bed was your *favourite ever*! That 'favourite' bed ended up becoming mine for the night as you stayed up until midnight watching Mummy's phone in ours!

### 1st June 2021

Lacking the requisite amount of sleep for a Little Man your age, you claimed you wanted to go back home. Pressed for a reason, you said that you were *missing Quartz!*

Driving out of the city we asked, 'Did you like Newcastle, Noah?' *No! We have been to the old castle!* Trying to explain our question felt pointless.

You grazed on snack after snack on the drive to Edinburgh and claimed you did not go to sleep because we were not travelling on a *big road*. I suppose we will have to start driving on motorways in order for you to nap!

Edinburgh Castle soared above where we parked our car. It must have been an imposing sight for a three-year-old and prompted a flurry of questions from you.

*Who lives there?*
*How old is the king?*
*Why did he die?*

None of which Mummy or I felt we could accurately answer without a lengthy Google search!

On Grassmarket we had lunch and played Dinosaur Snap. It is simply just not worth it to do anything other than give you enough time to shout *Snap!* when the cards are piled high. Whilst I am not as fully behind letting you win as your Mummy is, neither of us needed the emotional fallout that would have ensued whilst we were meant to enjoying ourselves on holiday!

The open-top buses caught your eye so we indulged in a hop-on, hop-off tour. Naturally, you wanted to sit on the top and enjoyed waving at people on the ground a lot more than your fellow passengers enjoyed you continually singing, *The roof! The roof! The roof is on fire!*

After difficulty getting you to sleep last night, we decided that Mummy would put you to bed tonight and I would go down to the bar to write this book. Only one winner there!

## 2nd June 2021

For two mornings in succession, I woke up on my own in the bed that was supposed to be yours! You claimed that the reason you climbed into our bed halfway through the night was because I did not give you a cuddle before you went to bed. I am pretty sure I did!

You often have difficulty responding immediately to instruction, which is to be expected at your age. Thankfully, the consequences could have been a lot worse when you ran off and got your arm stuck in a revolving door on the way out of the hotel!

The Covid-19 restrictions meant that we had to book to use the swimming pool when we arrived at the hotel yesterday. It was nice to see how your swimming has improved. Mummy is still not allowed to enter the swimming pool back home on a Saturday so it is difficult to monitor how you are developing. In comparison to Cornwall last summer, you are now really confident in the pool and did not want to get out.

The final leg of our road trip north was to Anstruther in East Fife, where we were staying with *our mate* Paul, who you know as Sucky, for four nights. Sucky has a dog like Harley, called Buddy, who you spent ages throwing a ball for in the back garden.

Now used to holidays in the United Kingdom, you referred to Sucky's house as *our holiday house* and could not understand why he was staying with us!

## 3rd June 2021

Your favourite saying at the minute is calling Mummy and I *a pesky meanine* whenever we do anything that you do not necessarily agree with.

Sucky was working so we went to the Scottish Deer Centre in Cupar. You loved feeding the different types of deer. You fearlessly fed some stags and some smaller deer, who left *deer snot* on your hand!

Your favourite animal was the Scottish wildcat but you were a bit wary of the bears, despite loving reading and singing about them.

You are developing confidence when playing with other children, which is a relief as so many kids have been affected socially and emotionally by the impact of living in lockdown. After lunch, we watched you approach two older boys and suggest they play hide and seek with you. You proceeded to count to ten and then ran up to one of the boys and shouted, *Found you!* even though he had not agreed to play!

I went playing golf with Sucky and Buddy at teatime and you stayed at his house with Mummy. Before watching *Shrek*, you had a shower with Mummy and *washed the baby* (Mummy's belly).

### 4th June 2021

Portugal was taken off the Green List which means that from 8th June people returning from holiday will need to self-isolate at home for ten days. Such unpredictability makes us feels vindicated in deciding to take another holiday in the United Kingdom, rather than go abroad.

When we asked what you wanted to do today you quickly responded, *Play golf with Daddy, Sucky and Buddy!* You evidently felt left out yesterday evening.

Sucky worked for an hour in the morning as he had to interview someone for a job. Whilst he was on the video call in his study, you burst through the door and asked, *Sucky?! Can you put* Paw Patrol *on the telly?* Hardly the experience the interviewee was expecting!

Later in the day, on the beach in St Andrew's, you were very interested in the rocks, rockpools, shells and other things you found lying on the sand. You found a dead, dried-up crab and innocently suggested that if we returned it to the sea it would come back to life.

We had been talking about how seagulls like to eat crabs and you witnessed first-hand how hungry the birds can get when one swooped down and stole a man's sandwich on the high street!

Sucky took you to a shop to buy your first putter. You then thought you could go on the eighteenth hole of The Old Course, the most famous golf course in the world, and play. So you could use your new putter freely we took you to the practice putting green at the driving range. You are very headstrong and did not listen to well-meant advice around your technique. *No! I can do it like this!* you insisted as you putted the balls into the deep pot bunkers rather than the holes!

There were 6,238 cases of Covid-19 recorded today, the highest daily total since mid-March. Is this a sign that people are becoming more relaxed during the summer months, tired of their lives being constrained for well over a year? Scientists are starting to strongly vocalise that removing social restrictions on 21$^{st}$ June is going to be too soon.

### 5$^{th}$ **June 2021**
You were three and a half years old today. Three years

ago on this very day we flew to Tenerife for ten nights on your first holiday abroad. Back then, it would have been impossible to predict the worldwide devastation that has since been inflicted by this virus.

After a lie-in you went to Anstruther Beach with Mummy, making up your own game of *stone cricket*. You were that engrossed that you refused to leave the beach, even after being offered an ice-cream.

You both joined me, Sucky and Buddy at Crail Golf Club for lunch. Predictably, you brought your new putter along. You really do get easily frustrated when you feel as though you cannot do something. I managed to prevent you from hitting chunks out of the practice putting green but could not stop you from throwing your new club in temper!

Watching the television back at the house you shouted for me to *come here!* I would not have turned to help you if I had known that your apparent emergency was you wanted a *bogey* out of your nose disposing of!

As I put you to bed, I asked you what the favourite part of your holiday had been. Your response? *Everything*. Bless you.

### 6th June 2021

*What?!* you barked, having not heard what Mummy said.

'Pardon', Mummy responded.

*Pardon?* you quizzically came back at her with.

This is a process we go through time and again in an attempt to instil decent manners in you.

You said that you were happy to go home because you had missed Quartz. Imagine all the fun that you would have missed out on had we done a U-turn in Newcastle-upon-Tyne five days ago?!

Your tablet entertained you for most of the long drive home. To be fair, it was only the second time you had watched it all holiday. It dawned on Mummy and I that we had just enjoyed our last holiday as a family of three. The next time we go away as a family, with your baby brother, there will be four of us.

**7th June 2021**
*But I am tired!* you moaned as we tried to get you up and ready for nursery.

You came home from nursery with a very good Progress Report. The pick of it for us was, 'Noah is fully toilet-trained but sometimes needs reminding when he is too excited with play'. We can certainly relate to that with the number of wet underpants we have changed since March last year!

Not listening to me when cleaning your teeth you jumped up banging my chin with your head, causing my top teeth to burst my bottom lip. You were very upset at the sight of blood in my mouth and were clearly very sorry!

**9th June 2021**
Our region, and one immediately neighbouring us, have been advised to reduce travel and contact with others due to the increase in the Indian variant of Covid-19.

Cases are on the rise, with 7,540 positive test results today. This is the highest daily total for over three months. Triggering the final stage of the 'roadmap' largely depends on the success of the vaccination programme. So far, 28.5 million people have received both doses of the vaccine, with 40.7 million people having had one dose. It is thought that 80% of the population have Covid-19 antibodies in their blood, either through being vaccinated or having contracted the virus.

### 10th June 2021

After asking you to get dressed, we were pretty sure we heard you say *Fucking hell!* as you turned away to go and do as you were told. We avoided asking you to repeat your retort, being mindful to be even more careful about what we say around you from now on. It is one thing using bad language but using it in context is an entirely different matter altogether!

Over 7,000 Covid-19 cases were reported for the second consecutive day, with 7 deaths.

### 11th June 2021

Mummy is now reaching the latter stages of her pregnancy. Kindly, you tell her that she *walks like a penguin* and do a pretty good impression of one yourself, waddling from side to side across the kitchen floor.

Mummy went out for her low-key baby shower with Stevie and some friends to celebrate the impending birth of your baby brother.

After nearly ripping your Euro 2020 wallchart in temper, you settled down with me to watch the tournament's opening ceremony, which was postponed last year due to Covid-19. The first game was played between Turkey and '*Tickly*' (Italy). I missed the first goal of the tournament as I struggled to find your *blue blanket* and favourite elephant teddy so you would go to sleep.

## 12th June 2021

I was away all day and night at Edgbaston in Birmingham watching England play cricket against New Zealand. This Test match was a Government Covid-19 test event where all 18,000 spectators had to display a negative lateral flow test on entry to the ground.

England's Test result was also negative, as we went on to lose by eight wickets very soon the following day.

The nightlife in Birmingham was somewhat subdued, having to remain seated at designated tables in bars and wear masks when walking around.

## 14th June 2021

'Freedom Day', the day when all restrictions on social contact are to be lifted, was originally scheduled for Monday 21st June. Today, the Government made the decision to push 'Freedom Day' back due to the Delta (Indian) variant of Covid-19 spreading too quickly. We are told that we will definitely be free from social restrictions on Monday 19th July. Are we confident this will be the case? We were told to prepare for a three-month lockdown in March 2020 and we are still in the midst of a pandemic.

I guess that I will have to continue writing this book for a bit longer!

## 16th June 2021 – 450 Days Since Lockdown Began

You have developed a couple of habits recently. The first is putting Mummy's hand cream on every time you have been to the toilet and washed your hands. Hand sanitiser has become an everyday staple of the Covid-19 diet. Following minor contact with others, it has become second nature to use the small, transparent bottles to squirt a liquid, which claims to kill 99.99% of bacteria, on one's palms. You have seen hand sanitiser on an abundance of occasions and have now progressed to using moisturiser!

A habit a considerably smaller number of people have inherited is saying the word *poop* constantly. You even like to form a little chain, *poop-a-poop-poop!* You sometimes combine this with turning around, parting your bum cheeks with your hands and 'blowing a raspberry' to mimic flatulence!

### 17th June 2021

Covid-19 cases are rising quickly across England, with infections increasing at a rate of 50% between 3rd May and 7th June. The current R rate is estimated to be at 1.44. The Delta variant has overtaken the Alpha (Kent) strain of the virus and now accounts for 90% of cases.

Having felt your baby brother kick for a number of weeks, your look of horror when you saw one of his limbs cause Mummy's tummy to bulge had us in fits of laughter!

### 20th June 2021

Whilst you did not refer to today, Father's Day, as 'Farmer's Day', you are still a bit confused about who the father is in our family. You did well to get it right in three guesses! You hid my presents around the house and set up a 'present hunt' only to then tell me where they were all hidden.

We went to a family day at Pontefract Racecourse where you had your first taste of betting on sport. You struggled to catch your breath as you dealt with the devastation caused by my horse pipping yours to the post in the first race. You certainly drew a lot of attention in the Picnic Enclosure as you cried, *It's not fair!* through snot and tears.

Luckily, you stuck with me for the next race and 'The Flying Ginger' gave you your first-ever winning bet! You enjoyed the novelty of using our money to bet on horses and tried to collect one set of winnings from the bookmaker! Not until you're eighteen, Little Man!

Chapter 21

# THE HOME STRAIGHT?

**21st June 2021**
Today was supposed to be 'Freedom Day', when social contact restrictions imposed by Covid-19 come to an end. When I started writing this book – 455 days ago – I, along with many others, naively felt that lockdown would only last for a couple of months. After a number of false dawns, millions of people still find themselves in a situation far removed from what they had been used to in their lives prior to the pandemic.

Will this be the last chapter? After what has occurred since 23rd March 2020, who knows?

**22nd June 2021**
England won their final game of the Euro 2020 group stage, beating Czech Republic 1–0 to finish at the top of Group D.

## 24th June 2021

Grandma Julie's sixty-first birthday.

You were sick in the night so we called nursery to let them know that you were not going in. The day brought back memories of the start of lockdown last year as Mummy and I were both working from home. Sat with us at the kitchen table, you practised using scissors, cutting holes in sheets of cotton. I tried to help your technique, which you did not favourably receive, shouting, *I don't like you!*

After lunch we dropped a chocolate cake at Grandma's for her birthday. You and I dropped Grandma and Grandad off at the train station and you were devastated that you were not allowed to go with them for the afternoon. Going out on the town when you are on the sick is widely frowned upon, Little Man!

Euro 2020 is in full swing and you now recognise England's national flag. Seeing a lot of these in the supermarket, you loudly announced, *We love England because they foul everybody!*

## 25th June 2021

Nana Roz kept you overnight at her house because Mummy and I went out for a meal with Auntie Stevie and Uncle Simon. When you found out that this was the plan, your bottom lip protruded as you meekly asked, *But who is going to look after my bunny?* Quartz feels an even bigger part of the family now that he has a cage inside the house.

Cases of Covid-19 continue to rise in all parts of the country. Nearly thirty-two million people have received both doses of the vaccine.

## 28th June 2021

The Government decided that lockdown would not end any earlier than Monday 19th July, ruling out the slim possibility suggested in reports this could happen on Monday 5th July.

Daily cases of Covid-19 are on the rise. More positively, the number of people dying from the virus is falling as a result of the successful vaccination programme. It is frightening to think where we would be were it not for the miracles performed by scientists.

In the Euro 2020 Round of 16, Spain beat Croatia 5–3 after extra-time and Switzerland beat France 5–4 on penalties, after a 3-3 draw, which meant that it was a record day for goals at any European Championship in history.

## 29th June 2021

You went to nursery in your clean, white England shirt and came home with it covered in stains.

England kicked off their Round of 16 tie against Germany at 5pm. You watched this at Grandma Buckley's as she did Mummy's hair, whilst I went to the pub.

England won 2–0 at Wembley, the first time they have beaten Germany in the knockout stages of a major tournament since the 1966 World Cup final, to make it through to the quarter-finals. A date with Ukraine awaits on Saturday.

There is a growing belief that England can go on and win a major tournament for the first time in fifty-five years.

## 30th June 2021

Last week at nursery, Darcie came into contact with a child

who subsequently tested positive for Covid-19. Today, Wednesday, was the sixth day of her weeklong isolation period.

You stayed at Grandma and Grandad's house last night and spent this morning with Grandad on your own. He took you to see how the building works were progressing at our new house and then to the country park. Grandad was waiting for you at the bottom of a slide that cascades down the hill, only to find out that you had taken yourself off to play with a group of little girls.

You are fully accepting of the fact that you will soon have a little brother. Before bed, in reference to you and I sometimes standing to share the same toilet bowl, you said to Mummy, *One boy, two boys, three boys! There'll be three boys crossing swords!* By the time your little brother can stand up to urinate, that might not be appropriate, Little Man!

The highest number of Covid-19 cases since late January, 26,068, was recorded today and fourteen people lost their lives. It feels as though it is hardly a situation that lends itself to being able to lead normal lives again in just over two weeks.

### 2nd July 2021

The sunflower you planted in Great-Nana Mave's garden is doing much better than the one that perished after a few days at home.

Due to a minibus mix-up at Mummy's school, we all had to drive it back after tea and park it in the school grounds. You were a touch disappointed that it was not an open-top or double-decker bus that Mummy had been driving on her school trip!

### 3rd July 2021

Last Saturday we should have gone to Ted's – or *Blackburn Ted* as you like to call your friend – house for his birthday party. It had to be pushed back to this afternoon due to Ted having to isolate after coming into contact with a child who tested positive for Covid-19 at school.

Having not been able to attend kids' parties properly for over a year, traditional games such as 'pass the parcel', are new to you. You did not win the main present but were more than pleased with the bag of sweets you got after unwrapping a layer of the parcel.

Despite not enjoying sitting down and watching football as much as you did when more entertaining things did not occupy your attention, you are certainly noticing the hysteria that is being whipped up by England's progress through the Euro 2020 tournament. You know the words to 'Three Lions' and 'Vindaloo' and sang along in the car journey home, yelling and pointing at every St George's flag you saw.

England beat Ukraine 4–0 in Rome, Italy, to make it through to the semi-finals against Denmark at Wembley Stadium on Wednesday.

### 4th July 2021

We finally managed to buy you an England flag after everywhere we looked yesterday had sold out.

Your baby brother is due to be born in five weeks' time so we got some stuff out of the loft to prepare for his arrival.

The building of the extension at the house we are moving to starts tomorrow so we need to think about putting our current house up for sale. You are anxious for confirmation that when we do move, we will be taking *the bunny*, the cushions and all of your toys with us!

## 5th July 2021

Boris Johnson will make England the most liberal society in Europe on 19th July, as far as Covid-19 restrictions are concerned. All that will remain will be the requirement to isolate for a week after a positive test, constraints on international travel as well as mandatory social distancing at airports and other points of exit and entry into the country.

Despite this good news, there are indications that we could be locked down again later in the year.

## 6th July 2021

Before bed last night you pulled the skin off a blister on your big toe. This morning, in your world, it prevented you from brushing your teeth, getting dressed for nursery or walking at all! You added even more fun to this drama when you took off all your clothes in the front room, claiming that you had wanted to get dressed yourself!

At the Wimbledon Tennis Championships there were full-capacity crowds on Centre Court and Court One. The largest sporting crowd, 60,000 people, since March last year was present at Wembley. Italy beat Spain 4–2 on penalties, after the game had finished 1-1 after extra-time, in the first semi-final of Euro 2020.

28,773 coronavirus cases were reported today, along with 37 deaths.

## 7th July 2021

'Three Lions' belted out from my car stereo as I dropped you off at Grandma and Grandad's. *It's coming home!* you shouted as you walked into their house, your St George's flag draped around your shoulders like a superhero's cape.

Making the most of Grandma and Grandad's train passes, you went for a day out. Darcie, bless her, was caught short in the park. Grandad's lyrical talent had you both giggling with hilarity when he came up with the following ditty:

'Darcie in the park,
Had a belly ache.
She couldn't find the toilet,
BLUP! Too late!'

We watched England's semi-final against Denmark at Grandma and Grandad's house. England conceded their first goal of the tournament to go 1–0 down. Before half-time, England equalised. You missed it live as you had gone into the kitchen to put your cup in the sink. You came running back into the front room, smiling, with your hands covering your ears, shouting, *It's so loud!* because everyone was cheering.

You went to bed at half-time as England won 2–1 in extra-time to make it to their first major tournament final since 1966.

They play will Italy, in the Euro 2020 Final, at Wembley in four days' time.

## 11th July 2021

The whole day was geared towards England's first ever appearance in a European Championship Final.

At Diddikicks, you labelled the red team *England* and the blue team *Italy*. Impressive, as neither Mummy nor I can remember telling you who England are playing in the final.

In the afternoon, we went to a 1950s-themed American diner with friends where there was an outdoor play area with a barn. You loved going down the slide with the bottom half of your body in a sack. At the bottom of a steep slide you had travelled down on my knee you said, *That made a tickle in my tummy!* Thankfully, you slept on the way home because we were in for a late night.

We watched the Euro 2020 Final in the golf club. England took a 1-0 lead inside three minutes, with Luke Shaw scoring the quickest ever goal in a European Championship Final. You were fascinated by everyone's celebrations, especially me running round going berserk!

Unlike other games throughout the tournament, you sat and watched large parts of the match. Your questions flowed.

*Foul! Why are there lots of fouls?*

*Why are we English? Are Italy 'Italish'?*

Italy equalised in the second half and the game went to extra-time and penalties. *Why's it taking so long to win the trophy?* England eventually lost 3-2 on penalties. *Why did we not win? Why did Italy win?* There was no simple answer to that, Little Man, but there was an overriding feeling that a golden opportunity had been passed up.

A reported 30.95 million people watched the match, which was more than the 27 million that watched Boris Johnson's 'Stay at Home' broadcast on that famous Monday evening back in March last year.

**12th July 2021**
The rain poured as I took you to nursery. 'It's a miserable day isn't it, Little Man?'

*But the flowers will be happy!* was your delightfully optimistic response!

You drew a beautiful family portrait today and walked around, proudly telling everyone, *I've drawn my Mummy really big. She's got a big, fat belly because she's got a baby!*

The Government confirmed that on Monday 19th July legal restrictions and social distancing related to Covid-19 will be lifted. However, this does not mean that the pandemic is over. Ambiguously, the Government is urging people to gradually return to normal. There is a nagging feeling that the 'normal' we knew more than eighteen months ago may never be a way of life again.

**13th July 2021**
It was 'Graduation Day' for you at nursery. You had a 'black tie' lunch and pictures with all your friends – Arthur, Isabelle, Jessica, Louis, AJ, Hazel, Phoebe and Jax. The latter is who you think we are naming your baby brother after!

**14th July 2021**
I took a day off work as Grandma and Grandad were away. I regretted not taking any in-car entertainment with us as you repeatedly asked, *Are we there yet?* on the way to Delamere Forest.

After a picnic, which consisted mainly of cold Margherita pizza for you, we went to look for the 'Gruffalo' in the forest. Filled with trepidation that we were going to come across a real 'Gruffalo', you were mightily relieved that it was only a wooden sculpture, enshrined by a metal fence so it did not become a breeding ground for Covid-19. Pointing at it, laughing with relief, you asked, *Why's it not real?*

In the middle of the woods you were caught short, claiming you needed *a wee and a poo*. We both got stung by nettles before I taught you how to squat and then covered your deed with ferns.

On the walk back to the car, much to your surprise, a pine cone fell out of a tree and landed on your head!

Manchester Airport's new Terminal 2 opened today so we stopped off at The Airport Pub on the way home. Playing on the aeroplane climbing frame, watching planes landing and taking off, made you want to go on a *big plane*. Then, in an innocent moment of resignation, you told a woman there with her grandchildren, *We cannot go on holiday 'cos of coronavirus.*

## 15th July 2021

You started at nursery the day you turned nine months old. Since then, your first nursery has closed down. You then temporarily moved to another one because of the pandemic. Ordinarily, today would have been your last day at private nursery until you start at school in September. To keep you in some kind of routine, and give Mummy a break, you will be doing the odd few days over the summer holidays. You went dressed as Spiderman for Superhero Day and took a card and a plant for each member of staff.

You came home with pictures of you and your friends,

and a poem from the staff. It was emotional reflecting upon the last three years and how much you have grown, learned and enjoyed education. To think that a pandemic has also been thrown into the mix made Mummy and I proud at how resilient you have been throughout all the changes.

Hopefully, on the few days you are attending over the summer, you will be able to say bye to your friends, none of whom are following you to your school nursery.

**16th July 2021**
Yesterday was Great-Nana Mave's birthday so you and Nana Roz took her out for lunch. You charmed the waitress into giving you an extra scoop of ice cream.

It was the last day of Mummy's school term – and Mummy's last working day until June 2022 – so she came home with lots of cards and presents for her and your baby brother. I was the only one who missed out, as Mummy's colleagues bought you a bubble wand!

The countdown to the arrival of your baby brother is now on. It is strange to imagine that, after everything we have lived through in this book as a family of three, there will soon be four of us.

**17th July 2021**
After swimming, you and Mummy went to the park for a picnic. Due to the scorching temperature, it was a race against time for you to eat your ice cream before it melted all over you!

Your Great-Uncle Ian was up from the south coast for the first time since December 2019. Lockdown has prevented him from making his trips north to see your Great-Nana Mave twice a year. As it was her birthday we all went out for a meal. You ate too many nachos for your starter so *Nana* James took you to feed the majority of your fish and chips to the ducks on the lake!

## 18th July 2021

Before Diddikicks, you were heartbroken that I had gone for a run without you. On my return, I asked if you wanted to run round the block to see the horses. After a slight pause, you answered, *Yes. But I'll just walk*, claiming you were actually too tired to run.

Later in the day, you pretended to help me and Grandad Col cut the hedge. As usual, you quickly became bored and chose to stand around, asking questions and accusing Grandad of making a mess as he sheared the leaves onto the footpath!

Collin Morikawa won The Open Championship at Royal St George's by two shots. 32,000 fans attended each day. Further signs, maybe, that we are edging back to normality.

Chapter 22

# FREEDOM AT LAST?

**19th July 2021**
Today had been billed 'Freedom Day' as social restrictions relating to Covid-19 were lifted. This meant that all legal constraints around mass gatherings have gone. We can all now attend weddings, funerals, concerts and sporting events without the number of people being limited. At midnight, nightclubs opened for the first time since March 2020.

The Government is still advising people to maintain a social distance and wear masks in public places. However, it is no longer the law.

The heatwave continued and you are not really enjoying the hot weather. Your breathing has been a bit shallow for the last few days so Mummy took you to see the doctor. All the way there you protested, *I'm fine*. It transpired that you thought you were on your way for more jabs! In the end, the doctor found nothing wrong with you.

Bedtime antics were taken to a new level when, watching our neighbour watering his plants, you got your knee stuck between the slats on your headboard. Mummy and I had to use some of our 'special cream' in order to free you!

## 21st July 2021

Soon, Wednesdays with Grandma and Grandad, as well as Fridays with Nana Roz and James, will be consigned to history when you start school nursery.

Today, Grandma and Grandad took you and Darcie to the beach at Lytham St Anne's. You loved going in the sea, digging in the sand and doing *bum bounces* on the trampolines.

When I picked you up, you immediately told me, *Darcie got into trouble for spitting her drink all over Grandma's car!* After I told you to stop 'telling tales', you denied you were, insisting, *It's true!* Haha!

## 22nd July 2021

Mummy took you to Hollingworth Lake with two of her friends from work, one of whom had a nine-week old baby girl. You were really good with the baby, tickling her feet and playing peekaboo.

You also took a keen interest in Mummy's friend breastfeeding, pointing at her and asking, *Is the baby hungry? Are those like udders?*

In the late stages of pregnancy, Mummy's feet are starting to swell. So, she was happy that you chose to go paddling in the lake, as opposed to walking round it.

**23rd July 2021**

Your baby brother is due in sixteen days' time so your car seat has been moved to *the big boy's side* of the car.

On the way to Legoland, my Father's Day present from you – Cheers, Little Man! – you commented, *This is the way to the airport*, after seeing the blue-and-white aeroplane signs on the motorway.

After ten minutes in Legoland, you told a member of staff, *I love it here!* There were some rides, Lego-building activities and a 3D cinema show, which was a new experience for you. In the shop, you bought your first Lego set with your unspent Christmas money.

The Tokyo Olympics got underway a year later than planned. Athletes will be competing in barren stadiums with strict Covid-19 protocols in place at all times.

**24th July 2021**

Despite Covid-19 restrictions being lifted, Mummy still cannot go into the swimming baths with you. We are not sure why.

Mummy took you to see Grandad Ste and Sharron and your great-grandparents, Anne and Mike, also turned up. You and Grandad sat silently on the couch for about fifteen minutes, concentrating on building your new Lego. I am very pleased that you have got the bug. It is much more difficult to get away with playing with plastic bricks when you do not have a three-year-old child as an excuse!

The nice weather continued so we went to a pizza barn and brewery. You kept saying, *But we can't eat pizza!* When questioned why, you explained, *'Cos it's from Italy!* The Euro 2020 final defeat evidently continues to cut deep.

### 25th July 2021

The atmosphere at Diddikicks felt more normalised, with several people being able to come and watch their children and adults not being required to wear face masks. The coaches have started to introduce an element of competition to the games which you really enjoy. You are very keen to point out when other children *cheat*!

We went to an event called 'Dino Land' in the afternoon. You ran around from dinosaur to dinosaur, which were life-size, moving models of different species, shouting out their names. Dinosaurs really are your specialist subject!

After standing in a queue for fifteen minutes to get your face painted, you decided that you did not want it done in the end! At the fairground, you 'braved' the dodgems and the rollercoaster. Mummy tried to go on the latter with you until being told that pregnant women could not ride, resulting in a 'toddle of shame' back down to the grass. The way you excitedly told Mummy about how much you had enjoyed yourself definitely contrasted with your anxious demeanour as the ride dipped and turned at fifteen miles an hour!

### 26th July 2021

Mummy dropped you off at the building site that will soon be our new home, as she had to go to the hospital to check that your baby brother was OK. You now know that he is going to be called Xander Joseph and it is a miracle you have not told anyone!

Xander was absolutely fine and you could see his pouting lips on the scan picture. Everyone is getting very excited to meet him!

It was Auntie Stevie's birthday so you and Mummy took her out for lunch. You promised to get her a cake to celebrate and the smallest one turned out to be big enough to feed the three of you!

### 27th July 2021

The number of new Covid-19 cases fell for the seventh continuous day. However, the 131 deaths as a result of the virus was the highest daily total since 17th March this year.

### 28th July 2021

All three of us have now got memberships at United which means that you will hopefully go to your first game at Old Trafford this season.

Talking about weddings and marriages with Grandma and Grandad, you and Darcie decided that it will be a good idea to get married to one another. Quizzed on this by me, you enthusiastically answered, *Because we love one another!*

### 29th July 2021

With Mummy being off work there was not a mad rush to get you into nursery. You did not see it this way and constantly told Mummy on the drive there, *We are late!*

On the way back to the car at the end of the day, you modestly announced, *Hazel loves me!*

### 30th July 2021

The Olympic Games is on the television every morning and you are taking an interest in sports such as swimming, canoe slalom and badminton. The novelty of it all is sending your inquisitiveness into overdrive.

*Why are there five circles?* in reference to the Olympic logo.

*Which one's England? Why is Blackpool Tower in Tokyo?*

Mummy and I went to a wedding so you spent the night at Nana Roz and James's house. Out and about in Nana Roz's car, you asked, *Why is there an Olympic sign on that Aldi van?*

All Covid-19 restrictions were absent at the wedding but we still had to wear masks when singing in church. Apparently, the virus is more likely to spread when people are belting out hymns!

**31$^{st}$ July 2021**
Having a BBQ, in all kinds of weather, has been the norm for us since the start of lockdown. Despite eating BBQ food throughout the pandemic, you have now decided that you do not like food with *black bits*. Getting you to eat proved a bit difficult at the BBQ we had been invited to.

At the same BBQ, you became overly frustrated that you could not tackle an eleven-year-old girl who plays for Blackburn Rovers. You really are a bit too hard on yourself at times!

**1$^{st}$ August 2021**
Mummy and I took you to Diddikicks together for the first time. Today was a 'Pirate Special' and you still hate these themed sessions. You called the warm-up, where the coach was pretending to be a pirate whilst dressed in his usual tracksuit, a *scary game*.

With Xander's arrival not too far away, each trip out feels like it could be our last as a family of three. I raised the seat on your balance bike in the park so that you could ride it properly. Mummy is not able to take you out on your bike alone now as you are too fast and she cannot keep you away from danger!

You have started to take more notice of road signs. Today, you were fixated on the 'No Stopping' signs in the park. *But why are them people stopping? But why has the ice-cream van stopped there?*

## 2<sup>nd</sup> August 2021

The last thing you want to hear from your three-year-old son first thing in a morning is, *But my willy's stuck up and won't go down!*

Mummy's friends from Blackburn came over for the day and you went to the park. You and *Blackburn Ted* played very nicely together.

The warm weather means that we like to keep the house ventilated. This has led to you becoming bothered about the accumulation of flies and other bugs inside. I brought you a Venus flytrap plant home so that your bedroom, at least, can be bug-free!

## 3<sup>rd</sup> August 2021

Overnight Stuart Bithell, who was in my year at school, won a gold medal at the Olympic Games in the men's 49er sailing.

You and Mummy met me at work during lunch, after you had been to minigolf, and we all went shopping for your nursery school uniform. You wanted to come back into my office with me, most probably remembering that the last time you were there you got fed some cake!

I had to come home early for the afternoon anyway because Mummy had to go to the hospital due to Baby Xander's movements reducing. Thankfully, everything was fine.

## 4th August 2021

You continue to enjoy watching the Olympic Games at breakfast. You are loving watching athletes compete in sports that you would not otherwise be interested in, or even know existed. Your enjoyment of the global sporting event taking place in Tokyo is such that you came running into the front room to me and announced, *If eating breakfast was a race, Mummy won gold and I won 'grey'* (silver).

In order to get you to brush your teeth properly, Mummy has introduced 'gold medal brushing'. This has worked to stop you from spitting your toothpaste into the sink as soon as your toothbrush enters your mouth.

For tea, we went to an Italian restaurant for the first time since the Euro 2020 Final. England's defeat on penalties obviously still hurts as you asked the waiter for an *English pizza*.

## 6th August 2021

This morning, it was the Olympic boxing that intrigued you as you could not work out why two people were hitting each other.

For the best part of nine months, you have appeared to have embraced the idea of having a baby sibling. So, it was a surprise to Mummy when she had the following conversation with you:

*I'm going to trip you up!*

'That's not nice... why would you do that?', Mummy responded.

*Because I don't want a baby!*

'Why?'

*Because I don't!*

This was strange considering how involved you have been choosing clothes and toys for Baby Xander, as well as kissing and hugging Mummy's belly almost every day.

As Mummy was reading you a bedtime story, you picked your nose and would have flicked the findings down the side of your bed if she had not intervened. You dirty tyke!

### 8th August 2021

Your baby brother, Xander Joseph Buckley, was due to be born today. The day came and went with no sign of his arrival.

It was the Closing Ceremony of the Olympic Games in Tokyo and Great Britian finished fourth in the medal table with sixty-five medals (twenty-two gold, twenty-one silver and twenty-two bronze).

Jason Kenny became the most decorated British Olympian of all time after winning a gold medal in the Keirin cycling event. This took his tally to seven gold and two silver medals.

You rounded off a fortnight of constant Olympic enquiries with, *Why did Kenny win? Why's he called Kenny?*

### 9th August 2021

The first time it happened you were forgiven for being a

three-year-old messing about. Patience and sympathy, especially from me, was in short supply when you got your knee stuck in your headboard for the second time in just over three weeks! This time, it took a bit longer to release you and panic certainly set in for me and Mummy. We are confident that the traumatic experience will stop you from doing this again!

### 10th August 2021

After nearly nine years living in our house, we put it up for sale.

Lionel Messi, who many say is the best football player of all time, left FC Barcelona to sign for Paris Saint-Germain after scoring 672 goals in 778 games for the Spanish club.

### 12th August 2021

Baby Xander continues to enjoy life in Mummy's tummy. He is now going to arrive later than you did at forty weeks plus four days. It feels weird waiting for him to arrive, knowing that our lives will never be the same again once he does.

### 14th August 2021

As Mummy bounced on her gym ball, *Why are you going on the ball? To bounce the baby out? OK. Bounce a bit higher!* was the sum of your enquiries, and subsequent advice, to Mummy.

United played their first game in front of a capacity crowd at Old Trafford for 524 days. They beat Leeds United 5–1, with Bruno Fernandes scoring a hat-trick.

Leaving the Thai restaurant where we had our tea, you held the palms of your hands together, whilst bowing at the waitresses saying, *Kop khun krap* (thank you)! The global number of cases of Covid-19 stands at 206,092,407, with 4,343,554 deaths.

**15th August 2021**
Grandma Julie came to Diddikicks for the 'Diddi Games', toddler football's take on the Olympics. You were very good at changing direction when dribbling and taking a touch before shooting. At the end of the session, you were so proud of yourself for winning a gold medal and failed to notice that every other child did too!

You spent all afternoon at Grandma and Grandad's whilst Mummy and I went for a walk to try and get Baby Xander moving. Last night, Mummy thought that she had started labour.

After you went to bed, Mummy started labour for real. At 11.25pm, Grandma and Grandad picked you up and you went to stay at their house. It would be the last time you went to sleep as an only child.

Chapter 23

# XANDER'S FIRST WEEKS

**16th August 2021**
At 12.35am, 1,350 days after you were born and 511 days since we were told to 'stay at home', Mummy gave birth to your little brother Xander Joseph Buckley. Xander was a shade over seven days late, and weighed seven pounds, five ounces.

We video-called you later in the morning and your first words on seeing Xander were, *He's so cute.* You then asked Mummy, *Are they putting your tummy back together?*

In the weeks leading up to Xander's birth, you had done so well keeping his name a secret. Now that he had arrived, you were insistent that his name was Ralphie.

From the hospital, Mummy and Xander went straight home and then I came to pick you up from Grandma and Grandad's. Your excitement had built across the day at the prospect of meeting your baby brother. You brought Mummy some flowers, a balloon and a card you and

Grandma had made. In it, you thanked me and Mummy for your baby brother.

On meeting Xander for the first time, referring to the red skin colour that newborn babies have, you asked, *But why is he so dark?*

All of our immediate family came to visit us before the day was out. You were even more animated than usual and loved all the presents you received for being a new big brother. Xander 'bought' you some Lego, which you were extremely pleased with. Taking turns at holding Xander, you and Darcie then treated him to a rendition of 'Happy Birthday'!

At bedtime, in what may become a frequent occurrence over the next few weeks, you emerged from your bedroom claiming, *I can't sleep because Xander's crying.*

Covid-19 has not disappeared from the news. People no longer have to self-isolate after coming into contact with someone who has tested positive for Covid-19 as long as they have received both vaccinations themselves.

### 17th August 2021

Your first morning as a big brother. It did not take long for the jealousy to set in. Walking into our bedroom, you saw Xander lying in between us on the bed. *But there's not enough room for me!* You are, however, taking a very loving interest in your baby brother. *Why's he crying? What is that thing on his belly button?*

Later on, Xander's nappy needed changing.

'Do you want to come and help Daddy change Xander's nappy?' I asked.

*Is it a poo or a wee?*

'A wee.'

In between that latter conversational exchange, and you arriving at the changing mat, Xander had decided to poo. In your very own accusatory tone, you whined, *You were joking! You tricked me!*

Sorry, pal. You will soon find out that babies are not so predictable!

**19th August 2021**

With Mummy breastfeeding Xander through the night, it is important that she gets some rest when she can. So, when you came into our room first thing in the morning, I took you and Xander downstairs.

It has not taken you long to become 'hands on', helping to change his nappy and feeding Xander his bottle. I made up a song, imaginatively named 'Lad Patrol' to the tune of the *Paw Patrol* opening track, in order to make any activities related to Xander fun.

You are doing really well adapting to Xander's arrival but, naturally, you are spending a lot more time with me. We went out for a drive to the pharmacy and the tip and you must have told me *I love you, Daddy!* at least six times! I am not going to forget you, Little Man!

We all watched *The Croods* in the afternoon, and I fell asleep with Xander. When I woke up, you were sat on the carpet sulking because it was not you I had cuddled dozing!

Later on, we paid Great-Grandad Mike and Great-Nan Ann a visit. Grandad Ste and Sharron were also there. This time, you actually sat on Great-Grandad's motorbike without getting scared. Despite it being stationary in the garage, you enthused, *It is so big and fast!*

**20th August 2021**

In the spirit of some Noah-Mummy bonding, you both made some 'Poisonous Warts', a recipe from your Gruffalo cookbook. Despite falling way short of winning a baking award anytime soon, they were much better than the 'Frog Muffins' you had both made previously.

Before Xander was born, Mummy had booked for me and you to go to a 'Jurassic Farm'. It was a great idea and, today, we spent the afternoon on tractor rides, watching shows and feedings animals. For you, there was also a bit of character-building involved as you tried to learn the art of being assertive. Two boys, at least a year older than you, kept pushing you off the bouncing pillow so I encouraged you to hold your own and get back on.

When we got home, I enquired as to why you keep saying you love me but do not replicate the same affection towards your Mummy. Your blunt response was, *I don't love mummies who've had babies come out of their tummies!* An extraordinary insight into the workings of a three-year-old's mind!

Xander's belly button clip fell off today.

**21st August 2021**

*Let me watch* Mighty Pups *on your bloody phone!*
'We don't say that word, Noah. Who have you heard say that?'
*Darcie.*

We are not too sure about that. Poor Darcie gets your blame for everything!

It is understandably a massive change for you, going from being an only child to a situation, overnight, where a very small person needs so much of your parents' time. It has not taken you long to develop a new range of attention-seeking behaviours, such as whistling, clicking your tongue and shouting *woo-hoo!* when you either need or want something.

## 22ⁿᵈ August 2021

Mummy left the three of us at home whilst she went for a bit of peace and quiet at the supermarket. Confusion set in when I asked, 'Shall we feed Xander in a minute?'

*With your boobies?* you responded, hilariously.

We all gave Xander his first bath and, like yours, this was in the bathroom sink. He did not enjoy it one bit, despite you trying your best to help by cupping handfuls of water into his face!

## 26ᵗʰ August 2021

Your last ever day at your private nursery school. You have attended there since September 2019, when the first one you went to closed down. Shamoona, or *Shami* as you have always called her, gave you a cuddle as you left for the last time and told you she loved you. Mummy was in tears of emotion when she picked you up with Xander. You said that you had missed Xander, gave him a kiss and stroked his face. You are certainly learning how to be gentle with him.

I went to watch the Test match between England and India at Headingley Cricket Ground in Leeds. For reasons only known to you and your three-year-old mentality, you refused to speak to me when I video-called home to speak to you and Mummy!

**27th August 2021**

As I left home to go and work with Grandad Col at our soon-to-be new home, you stood at the front door in floods of tears because you wanted to come with me.

After going for lunch with Mummy, Nana Roz and Great-Nana Mave, you called by at the house to see how we were getting on. The fire burning all the old kitchen and bedroom units in the back garden caught your attention and you were confused as to why no one was ringing the fire brigade!

United announced that they had reached an agreement with Juventus for Cristiano Ronaldo to return to the club, more than twelve years after he had left for Real Madrid.

**28th August 2021**

Long before the world knew anything of the virus that has dictated our lives for the best part of eighteen months, me and Uncle Liam took you and Darcie to Trentham Monkey Forest. For a child with such a fantastic memory, it was surprising that you did not remember going there previously as we walked through the entrance gates today.

Even more surprising was that we bumped into Birchy, Matilda and Theo who were camping with family in nearby Stafford. *Why is Birchy's holiday house a tent?* was a question you were keen to get answered.

The forest is full of barbary macaque monkeys roaming freely. You were worried that they were going to pinch Xander, who more or less slept the whole way round the forest, from his pram.

**29th August 2021**

The extent to which you are helping with Xander seems to

stretch each day. Now, you insist it is your job to make his bottles on the Tommee Tippee machine. You are clearly enjoying being a big brother.

I am getting annoyingly good at not qualifying for the showpiece event of the year at the golf club, the Captain's Final, so I caddied for Grandad Col instead. You and Darcie were standing on the busy balcony as we walked up the eighteenth hole. Darcie appeared very pleased to see us but you were sulking because you wanted to play on the eighteenth green!

**30th August 2021**
*But I'm your Little Man, Mummy!* you reminded her after hearing her use your moniker when talking to Xander!

A few weeks after you were born, we took you for a newborn photoshoot. This morning, it was Xander's turn. Only he had you, his big brother, with him on some of his shots. You did really well and seemed to enjoy being in front of a professional camera lens!

You have started to pretend Xander can speak, putting on a squeaky voice and saying, *I love you, big brother!* There's a narcissist in you somewhere!

Auntie Stevie tested positive for Covid-19. Despite having had both vaccinations, she still felt really ill from the effects of the virus.

**1st September 2021**
You and Darcie both start nursery, full-time, in different primary schools on Monday 6th September. This means that today was the end of an era as far as spending regular Wednesdays with Grandma and Grandad are concerned.

You managed to combine what have grown to become yours and Darcie's favourite activities. A chippy lunch, ice cream and a visit to the park.

Mummy and I went into Manchester to do some shopping and have lunch. In the shops, the low levels of stock on the shelves was evidently stark. Covid-19 has had an impact on imported goods being able to get into the country on a regular basis.

Cristiano Ronaldo became the leading international goalscorer of all time, scoring his 110$^{th}$ and 111$^{th}$ goals, in Portugal's 2–1 win over the Republic of Ireland.

**2$^{nd}$ September 2021**

Your little brother Xander became official as we went to register his birth at the town hall. The Covid-19 restrictions meant that Mummy had to do this alone whilst you and I stayed in the car.

Car journeys are now filled with Word Association and a game you and Mummy play, which goes a bit like this:

*Mummy... I love you to the moon and back.*

'I love you to the sun and back.' You, saying whatever you see out of the window, *I love you to the fire station and back.*

'I love you to the car park and back.' And so on. I am sure this is as annoying to read as it was for me to listen to!

Your brazen cheekiness was evident when you responded to Mummy's request for you to go upstairs and get ready for bed by saying, *No! Not when Mummy says! When Daddy says!* There is certainly a fine line between having bundles of character and pushing boundaries, as well as your Mummy's patience.

Almost inevitably after Auntie Stevie's positive test, Uncle Simon now also has Covid-19.

### 3rd September 2021

Xander was asleep when we set off to play minigolf at Dino Falls. He was still asleep over four hours later after we had been to Pizza Hut for a buffet lunch.

On one hole you beat both of us by getting a two, compared to the threes we could only manage. You got a touch upset when Mummy hit her ball into the *lava*, as you thought it was going to melt. You missed Mummy's hole-in-one on the last hole because you were preoccupied that your ball had *gone forever* after disappearing down the drainpipe which stops people from playing again for free!

You thought that the Pizza Hut buffet was great because you did not have to sit still for long before you went back for more pizza and pasta. Unlike at home, there was no expectation that you ate your crust. I explained, 'It is an all-you-can-eat buffet, Noah. We don't fill up on crust', before looking you in the eye, pointing at my temple and saying, 'Tactical'. Focusing on the last word of that particular sentence, you queried, *Daddy? Why did you say testicle?* Yet another innocently priceless moment!

Before bed, at your request, we re-enacted the opening scene from the Disney animation film, *The Lion King*. I was cast as Rafiki the mandrill and Xander was Simba the lion cub. You were very amused as I lifted Xander, arms outstretched, with the song 'Circle of Life' belting out from Alexa!

**4ᵗʰ September 2021**

Over the past few days you have not really been yourself. You have been tired, lacking an appetite, irritable and more emotional than usual. You denied feeling unwell but this morning you came out with a rash on your hands, feet, mouth and tongue. It did not take a doctor to diagnose you with hand, foot and mouth disease.

Hand, foot and mouth disease is more contagious for children. Therefore, we had to keep you away from kissing and touching Xander. Obviously, this made you want to kiss and touch Xander more! Mummy would have kept you from going swimming, if she had remembered that it was back on in the first place!

**5ᵗʰ September 2021**

Diddikicks was very busy and borderline chaotic. It is quite clear that you have outgrown the group and I have been looking at where else there is for children your age to play football. You do enjoy it, but often lose concentration because of how repetitive the sessions are. Today, you fell into a wall after daydreaming whilst rolling the ball under your foot!

Great-Nan Ann and Great-Grandad Mike called round to our house for some lunch. Great-Nan Ann had a brain operation a few years ago which means she is forgetful and becomes easily confused. It is sad because she cannot remember us visiting her house a few days after Xander was born.

The pizza barn is fast becoming our favourite place to go and we took advantage of the late summer heatwave. You played football on the grass with Mummy and when she scored you told her, *You have got to slide on your knees like Bruno!*

Mummy spent the day becoming intermittently emotional at the thought of you starting school nursery tomorrow. Time has flown by and we can still clearly remember when you were just three weeks old like Xander.

We have gone through a period of significant change over the last few months and you have coped really well. Starting school nursery tomorrow will be another big step for you. We can tell that you are unsure about going so we spent time reassuring you that you will be fine and you will actually love it!

After going to bed, I came upstairs to find you asleep on the carpet in the doorway to your bedroom. Maybe you were too tired to escape?

### 6th September 2021

Back to work for me and, more importantly, your first day at school nursery. We are going to apply for you to enter the reception class in twelve months' time so it was, in effect, your first day at school. We tried to match your apprehension with enthusiasm as you kept saying, *I don't want to go to school!*

You spoke on separate video calls to Grandma Julie and Darcie whilst putting on your new uniform. Seeing how excited Darcie was did not distract you from your negative perception of how the morning was going to go. You were adamant that Mummy was going to take you into the classroom for five minutes and then bring you home!

The plan was for Mummy to take you in and for me and Xander to wait outside, as per the original Covid-

19-related instructions back in June. However, we were all allowed in and you were soon playing with bricks, vehicles and dinosaurs and left to enjoy your first morning at school nursery.

You had a great first day, receiving stickers for good sitting, looking, listening and tidying up! You went to Nana Roz's for lunch so that she could see you in your new uniform.

After three weeks of a largely unstructured routine, you had a bath and went to bed at a relatively early time. Xander is your latest excuse for not settling and constantly getting back out of bed. An hour after we had turned off your lights, you came to the top of the stairs and shouted, *Calm Xander down because I can't get to sleep with that noise!*

Covid-19 has certainly not disappeared, although its prevalence in daily news articles has dropped significantly since 'Freedom Day' on 19th July 2021. The build-up to Xander's birth, and the weeks that have followed, have shifted our focus inwards onto the significant changes in our family.

That is not to diminish the pain and suffering so many people continue to endure. Despite having several vulnerable people in our family, we are so lucky not to have lost anyone close to us. Sadly, the same cannot be said for millions of families around the world.

On 6th September, 41,192 people tested positive for Covid-19 in the United Kingdom. Forty-five people also died from coronavirus. Since 31st August, 263,885 positive cases have been reported. This represented an increase of 12.2% on the seven days which preceded it. In the same period, 789 people died. Encouragingly, the number of daily deaths is falling, possibly as a result of the groundbreaking vaccination programme rolled out across the country.

The Government continues to stress the importance of using face coverings, observing social distancing and making sure that all indoor spaces are as ventilated as they can be. It is easy to become complacent, having lived in a constrained manner for so long. However, Covid-19 is still here.

From 10$^{th}$ September, the following changes are being introduced as the rules are relaxed further. Up to fifteen people, from four households, will be able socialise in a family home. A requirement for table service in restaurants and bars has been the norm ever since they first reopened in July 2020. However, customers will be able to go to a bar to order, and pay for, food and drinks. Inside, customers will still need to sit at their table and will not be allowed to drink standing up. Outside, due to the lowered risk of Covid-19 transmission, customers will be able to stand.

At live performance events indoors, people will no longer have to buy a ticket in advance. However, they must still sit down and provide their contact details through the NHS Track and Trace app. Guests at weddings will be able to dance, which has not been the case previously.

For millions of people used to being office-based, working from home full-time has become a way of life. Many people are anxious about returning to the office. I feel as though people's working patterns will never return to how they were pre-Covid-19. The impact of the pandemic will continue to reverberate down the years given the profound effect it has had on employment, family and social relationships, as well as the physical and mental health of hundreds of thousands of people.

Chapter 24

# PLAN B AND THE RISE OF OMICRON

There was never an end date in mind when writing this for you, Noah. The journey through this pandemic has been unpredictable, to say the least. Covid-19 has succeeded in saturating people's daily lives for longer than anyone could have imagined. Coronavirus has consumed news bulletins and occupied the consciousness of almost everyone on the planet.

Where is the end? Will there ever be an end? Where is a fitting moment to draw a line in the sand and move on from such a momentously devastating period of modern history?

By 9th September, more than ninety-two million doses of the Covid-19 vaccine had been administered in the United Kingdom. Public Health England estimated that more than 100,000 deaths were prevented as a direct result of the vaccination programme. It is scary to think about where we might have been were it not for the development, and subsequent success, of the vaccines.

On 14th September, the Government announced their Plan B. This was their strategic response should infection rates rise again throughout the autumn and winter. It is vital that the NHS is not placed under such weight of pressure again. Reverting to Plan B will mean having to work from home unless impossible to do so. It will mean wearing face masks indoors and requiring proof of having had both doses of the vaccine, through the NHS Covid Pass, when entering large, organised crowds. Imposing Plan B's regulations will be used to slow the spread of the virus, relieve the NHS of any unnecessary pressure and allow time for more doses of the booster vaccination to be made.

On 16th September at 1.48am, your cousin Ralphie Thomas Buckley was born, weighing seven pounds, fourteen ounces. Darcie was absolutely thrilled to have a baby brother, certainly not bothered about continuing to be alone as the only little girl in our family.

On 16th October, Nana Roz and *Nana* James finally tied the knot. Mummy was a bridesmaid and you a page boy, which extracted even further emotion from her as you both walked down the aisle. Imitating my method of attracting people's attention as Master of Ceremonies, tapping your wine glass with a spoon led to it ending as a shower of shards on the floor!

On 26th November, the World Health Organisation identified the Omicron strain of coronavirus to be of concern. Omicron quickly became the most common variant of the virus worldwide. Researchers suggested that Omicron was more easily spread because it can infect people even if they have received both Covid-19 vaccinations.

On 8th December, Boris Johnson announced that the

country was adopting Plan B. Omicron had won. This was almost certainly the right call. On 21$^{st}$ December, it was estimated that 1.9 million people in the country were infected with Covid-19. This was double the number of people who had the virus back on 5$^{th}$ September.

Chapter 25

# WHEN COVID CAME HOME

**21st December 2021**
Whilst pork roasts are not my favourite it still came as a surprise, when eating one Mummy had made, to realise I could not taste the mash, carrots or anything else on my plate.

*I can't taste anything either*, you claimed, trying to get out of eating your tea!

Loss of taste is a symptom of Covid-19. However, the lateral flow test I took at home came back negative.

**22nd December 2021**
The NHS advice is to go for a PCR test if you have symptoms of Covid-19, or if you return a positive lateral flow test.

The temporary testing centre, set up in the car park of the leisure centre where you play football, had not gone unnoticed by you. *Near Diddikicks?* you asked as I left the house early in the morning to go for a test. I then had to work my last day before Christmas at home, and isolate, until the result of my test came back.

You went for a walk around the lake with Mummy and Xander. You encouraged Mummy to take you to the café, as opposed to picking up some chips to take away, because you wanted to get warm.

The more contagious Omicron variant of Covid-19 resulted in more than 100,000 cases, 106,122 to be exact, being recorded today. This is the first time daily case numbers have exceeded five figures since the start of the pandemic.

### 23rd December 2021

At teatime, 638 days since we went into lockdown, our household recorded its first positive Covid-19 test. Remarkably, given the events of the previous two days, this belonged to Mummy! She found out after taking daily lateral flow tests as I awaited my test result.

Five minutes later, I received my PCR test result via text message. Unbelievably, it was negative. This meant that Mummy had to stay at home for at least seven days. I was allowed to go out as long as my daily lateral flow tests returned a negative result.

This meant that we would have to spend Christmas Day at home as a family of four. I quickly jumped in the car and went to the supermarket to buy everything we would need for Christmas dinner!

119,789 cases were recorded today, a worrying increase on yesterday's record number.

## 24th December 2021

This morning it was Mummy's turn to go for an early PCR test.

In preparation for the last Christmas in our house, you helped me *make the turkey*. This was what you called mixing the marinade and spreading it all over the skin.

In the afternoon, I took you and Xander to Grandma and Grandad's. The 'Christmas Elf' had delivered some presents for you both in a large gift bag. I asked if you had been 'Naughty', 'Nice' or 'I Tried', the three choices on the bag from your grandparents, and you honestly declared the latter!

After tea, you and Xander opened your Christmas Eve boxes and we all put our Christmas pyjamas on. You failed to notice that yours had been recycled from last year as they still fit.

After watching *Mickey's Christmas Carol – That was a short film* – and leaving milk, a mince pie and a Celebrations chocolate for Father Christmas, as well as a carrot and reindeer food at the back door for Rudolph, it was time for bed.

## 25th December 2021

You must have tried hard enough to be a good boy this year because Father Christmas did make a stop at our house.

Despite the front room being stacked with presents, the first thing you did was find one of mine and announce it was a dartboard! Opening all of yours, and Xander's, presents took that long you had to break for breakfast. Your favourite toy was a Hot Wheels shark from Nana

Roz and you chose to bring that to the pub with Xander and I.

It was sad that Mummy had to stay at home and isolate, but she did not want Covid-19 to break our family tradition of a few drinks before Christmas dinner.

For our family dinner, Xander sat at the table with us, his chair on the buffet, and you made him wear a paper hat. In spite of Mummy's positive Covid-19 test, it was nice to relax and enjoy the day together. It is miraculous that it has taken so long for any of us to have to isolate and, thankfully, no one is seriously unwell.

For the rest of evening, Mummy and I played with you and your new toys. I quite liked that you left me to build your Lego without too much interference affecting my concentration.

So, that was the story of Xander's first Christmas. I wonder how many years it will be before we are alone as a family of four on Christmas Day again?

## 26th December 2021

Mummy awoke to text message confirmation that she had tested positive for Covid-19. Not anything unexpected. Her festive isolation continued so it was my responsibility to get you out of the house to burn off some energy.

At the tip, you were more interested in asking questions about the place than you were in putting cardboard where I had asked you to put cardboard.

*What goes in there? Why aren't we going over there? What's that digger doing?*

The purpose of our trip to the park afterwards was for you to prove to yourself that you can glide and balance on your bike. This is before we introduce your new pedal bike with no stabilisers. You did not know that but you certainly did not lack confidence, weaving in and out of dog walkers and stopping yourself from riding into bushes.

As you were falling asleep eating your spaghetti bolognese at 6.30pm, Mummy and I chatted about the possibility you also had Covid-19. You had complained of a headache throughout the evening. When you were asleep in bed, Mummy put a swab up your nose. This confirmed that you did indeed have coronavirus.

## 27<sup>th</sup> December 2021

The tiring effects of the virus meant that you slept for over fourteen hours. When you woke up, you told us that your headache had gone.

*Why?* you asked worriedly, when we broke the news to you that you had Covid-19. The fact that Mummy also had it, and was not unwell, reassured you somewhat. Xander, who has a cough and is sleeping more than usual, has probably got the virus too but we cannot confirm this as the swab will not fit up his tiny nostrils!

So, that means that Mummy has to stay in until at least 30<sup>th</sup> December and you until 2<sup>nd</sup> January 2022. Therefore, your trip to the park with me was your last excursion of the year.

Xander is a very smiley baby, but he does not make much noise. You have made it your mission to try and make him giggle. He does find you funny but inadvertently encourages you by smiling at you when you are being cheeky to us!

## 28th December 2021

*What's the plan today?* you asked Mummy, not quite fully understanding how a Covid-19 quarantine works.

After my negative lateral flow test, I took Xander to do some sales shopping. You watched *Mia and Me* on Netflix, a programme that Mummy has had little choice but to become invested in with you. Being the comedian I am, I brought you and Mummy a 'Get Well Soon' card home!

Not being able to leave the house is leading to you becoming quite demanding. It must be difficult for you, as a four-year-old, to understand why you cannot go anywhere when you are not really ill. I played on your constant requests for service and attention by calling you Your Majesty. This joke wore rather thin very quickly and, at bedtime, you growled back at me, *I'm not Your Majesty! I'm your Little Man!*

## 29th December 2021

Yesterday, the country recorded a record 117,093 positive Covid-19 cases, which broke the previous record of 113,628 set on Christmas Day.

Still returning negative lateral flow tests, I went back to work and it was left to Mummy to entertain you all day. Receiving lots of new presents two days before you got Covid-19 was extremely good timing!

Your imagination has started to run a bit wild at bedtime. After being in bed for a short while, you came to the top of the stairs worried about monsters, foxes and other people being in the house. Mummy managed to get you back in bed but, minutes later, you woke up heartbroken about Marble, our rabbit who was taken too soon.

*But I miss Marble! Why does Marble live in the hills? But why am I not going to see Marble again?!*

Mummy got in bed with you, stroked your nose and sang nursery rhymes until you fell asleep.

### 30th December 2021

The Omicron variant of Covid-19 is much more contagious than, but not as potent as, previous strains. The symptoms are similar to those of the common cold.

With you and Mummy testing positive for Covid-19, and me having a cold in the run-up to Christmas, we assumed that you had both caught it off me. Today, that theory was dispelled when I also tested positive for Covid-19. *Come, Daddy! I'll show you why you have got Covid. Look! Two lines*, you declared, pointing at the plastic test, almost triumphantly!

Being confined to the house is sending you crazy, not being able to burn off all your energy. You have self-diagnosed yourself with *cabin fever*.

### 31st December 2021

A total of 12,395 people are currently in hospital with Covid-19. This is the highest number since 25th February. Will this pressure on the NHS force another lockdown? It certainly feels like we know of more people who have had coronavirus in the last few weeks than at any other point throughout the pandemic.

You helped us make tapas for our last meal of the year. We made seven different dishes and when we asked which one was your favourite, you held a piece of bruschetta aloft and announced, *this!*

At 8pm, you watched the firework display from Abu

Dhabi on the television and went to bed wishing us a *Happy New Year!*

Mummy and I went to bed before midnight on New Year's Eve for probably the first time this century. The holiday season has been a strange one, so it did not really come as a surprise.

As we enter the fourth calendar year of coronavirus's existence, it is difficult to remember what it was like before Covid-19 because an immovable feature of everyday life. Back in autumn, it felt as though we had managed to shrug of coronavirus. Now, it has returned to pervade our lives in a bigger way than at any other point since the start of the pandemic.

Thankfully, the Omicron variant is not as deadly as previous Covid-19 strains. As a family, the symptoms have only manifested themselves through headaches, tiredness and coughs.

Reflecting on the predictions made a year ago, our family is now complete with the addition of Xander Joseph. Our Little Xan, we dare not call him Little Man, or *Troublemaker* and *Little Monkey*, as you like to call him, could not have fitted into our lives any better. The love that you have for each other is clear, and something to be treasured. Watching Xander's face light up with a smile when he hears your voice is priceless. It is clear that the foundations for a precious, lifelong relationship have been laid.

The house move and family holiday abroad did not materialise in 2021. Over the course of the next few weeks, we will bid farewell to the home Mummy and I have lived in for over nine years and move a little over a mile down the road.

The project on the new house has not been without its issues but we hope that, once we move, it will be a home where you and Xander enjoy a wonderfully happy childhood.

A holiday to Gran Canaria for a fortnight is also on the horizon. There have been many false dawns during this pandemic. We hope there will not be any more Covid-19 restrictions imposed to prevent us from going. It will be Xander's first holiday abroad and the first for you in more than half your lifetime.

Happy New Year, Little Man, and, of course, Little Xan.

### 1st January 2022

New Year's Day. With your school holidays turning out to be a series of overlapping isolation periods all the days feel to have merged into one. Your New Year's resolution was to *play games* and that is exactly what you did all afternoon.

Mummy's isolation period ended a few days ago so she took Xander shopping. I took a lateral flow test which came back negative so, later in the afternoon, we went for a walk being sure to stay away from anyone else. I asked you not to stand in a puddle because it looked as though it contained poisonous mercury and your response was, *But my wellies cannot drink!* You are too clever for your own good!

A record high 162,572 positive Covid-19 cases were recorded today. The daily numbers are just staggering. In other news, it was the warmest New Year's Day on record, with the temperature reaching 16.2°C in St. James's Park, London.

## 2<sup>nd</sup> January 2022 – 650 Days Since Lockdown Began

*I'm allowed out!* you shouted as soon as you woke up! Your isolation period was over and you definitely knew it! You celebrated by going to mini golf with Mummy and Xander. I stayed at home.

Having recorded a negative lateral flow test for the second day running, I went to a drive-thru PCR test centre to find out for certain whether or not I had Covid-19.

Xander usually reserves his tricks and noisy moments for when you are in bed but this afternoon he rolled over for the first time. At teatime, after constantly flicking your baby brother on the nose and refusing to stop, your sticky toffee pudding was kept in its packaging. Cue tears, snot and a verbal outburst aimed at me. *You meanie! I'm never playing with you again!* This was very quickly retracted when, twenty minutes later, you asked me to help build your marble run. *I was only joking*, you meekly claimed.

## 5<sup>th</sup> January 2022

Back to school for you. Grandma gave your hair an overdue trim yesterday and you now think that you look like your friend Finley from your class.

The day after my visit to the drive-thru testing centre, my PCR test came back positive. Now in my sixth day of isolation, I am still testing positive for Covid-19. Picking up my positive lateral flow test from the kitchen worktop, you enquired, *Who's still got Covid?* Knowing what a positive test for a deadly virus looked like was something I never had to get to grips with when I was four years old!

Mummy made sure she stocked up on mince pies

when she went shopping to feed your addiction which lingers on from Christmas.

### 6th January 2022

Running into our bedroom first thing in the morning, you shouted, *Come and look in my bedroom! You will never believe it!* Pointing outside at the snow you suggested, *I think it is Christmas again!* Disappointingly for you, Little Man, it is not.

Thinking ahead to our house move, you were eager to ensure that your sticker charts, of all things, moved with us.

We applied for your primary school place. Hopefully, the application will be successful and you will move up to the reception class in September.

### 7th January 2022

My lateral flow test was finally negative. However, as yesterday's was not, I am not officially allowed to leave the house until tomorrow.

You were not in Mummy's good books after she picked you up from nursery. First, you shouted at her in the car because she could not hear you. Calling her *ugly* when you got home was also not a great move. Oops!

### 8th January 2022

My isolation period finally ended. This concluded sixteen days over Christmas and New Year where at least one of you, Mummy or I could not leave the house.

You went to see Grandad Ste and Sharron with Mummy, Xander and Stevie to swap Christmas presents.

On walking through the front door, you immediately asked, *Are we opening our presents then?*

Xander is teething so he spends quite a lot of the time trying to gnaw off his thumb!

As of today, 150,057 people in the United Kingdom have died within twenty-eight days of testing positive for Covid-19.

### 9th January 2022

Mummy, Grandma and Auntie Emma went to a spa for the day so parenting responsibilities were left to Grandad Col and me.

The day got off to a painful start. You ended up with a bruised eye after sliding into a chair at Diddikicks and then bit your tongue eating McDonald's at lunch.

We had fun in the park. You pushed your scooter down the hill and chased after it. We, along with strangers, were in hysterics when you fell in the mud. Undeterred, you got up to continue running after your scooter, your tracksuit bottoms sliding slowly down to your ankles with every stride.

Auntie Alice had joined us in the park so Uncle Kyle met us all for tea at our favourite Chinese restaurant. Duck is now your favourite food and you devoured more than your allocation of pancakes!

As we were leaving I heard you shout, *Uncle Aaron!* Checking that that it was definitely my attention you wanted, I turned to see you on all fours on the bench next to the bar with your bare bum exposed! Admittedly, it was very difficult to keep a straight face as I verbally reprimanded you for gross public indecency!

**11<sup>th</sup> January 2022**

We received confirmation from the solicitors' office that the sale of our family home will go through on Friday 28<sup>th</sup> January. Exciting stuff, although we are not sure where we will be living after then if our new home is not ready to move in to!

Today marked one hundred days since I last had an alcoholic drink so you kindly bought me a card and some sweets. Holding the bag of sweets, as you approached me walking into the house from work, you suggestively asked, *But you share, don't you, Daddy?*

**12<sup>th</sup> January 2022**

Brushing your teeth you innocently enquired, *What do you want to do today, Daddy?* as though I had any choice other than to go to work.

Xander went to Grandma and Grandad's for the day to give Mummy a chance to continue boxing things up for the house move. Xander's teeth are still troubling him to the point where he is now blowing raspberries. *Xander the Panda-fish* is the new name you have for your little brother.

News continues to leak that Members of Parliament attended parties at Westminster during the early stages of the first lockdown. There are calls for Boris Johnson to resign. Admittedly, it has been difficult to adhere to the lockdown restrictions at times, and people have bent the rules to breaking point. However, for figures of authority to be partying in the formative stages of the pandemic felt hypocritical beyond belief when thousands of people were succumbing to the virus.

**14th January 2022**

Working from home, I received the awful news that my childhood friend Shaun had died. Growing up, I was best friends with his younger brother Matt. As a child, Shaun was the closest thing I had to a big brother. We have many happy memories of hours spent playing football on the park, pretending to walk out to represent United at Old Trafford in the UEFA Champions League.

It is tragic that someone who was always smiling, joking and willing to stop for chat can, deep down, feel incredibly sad. Shaun had so many people who loved and cared for him and his passing will undoubtedly be felt far and wide. You met Shaun once as we were driving out of the car park at Diddikicks and we sang a few United songs with him.

Your bad day for failing to listen at nursery was compounded by the fact that you 'stole' a tennis ball and brought it home in your bag. You cried after Mummy, somewhat harshly in my opinion, told you that little boys who steal get taken to jail by the police! You drew a 'picture of apology' for your nursery teacher, which you are going to take in on Monday morning.

For the last few weeks, you and I have been learning Spanish on the Duolingo app in preparation for our holiday to Gran Canaria. All week this, as well as your bedtime story, has been taken away from you as punishment for continuing to wee in your pants. Tonight, you went one further and pooed in them. What's going on, Little Man?

**16th January 2022**

Xander was five months old today. His teething is causing

his bottom jaw to move from side to side as though he has taken an illicit substance.

You helped me take some rubbish from our new house to the tip. Whilst at the house, you complained that your play room is *too small* and said that you wanted to share the front room with me and Mummy instead!

In sport, England lost The Ashes 4–0 in Australia to cap off a miserable winter of cricket.

In tennis, the men's world number one Novak Djokovic was deported from Australia ahead of the Australian Open for failing to comply with the entry rules around Covid-19. To travel to Australia, you either have to be vaccinated or prove evidence that you have not been due to medical reasons. Djokovic met neither criteria which means that he cannot compete for a record twenty-first Grand Slam title.

**17th January 2022**

As you sat quietly in Mummy's car on the way to nursery, clutching your 'picture of apology', she asked, 'What are you thinking about, Noah?' *Not stealing*, you mumbled back.

Happy Monday!

**18th January 2022**

Despite claiming that it is *tricky* being well-behaved, you had a really good day at nursery. Your behaviour was credited with an appearance on the 'Happy Board' and you were taken to see the headteacher for showing 'caring behaviour'.

You still go to bed every night with your dark-blue

muslin cloth. You covered Xander with it, telling him, *I had this blanket when I was your age.* You are four, Little Man, not forty-four!

## 19th January 2022

After work, I went with Grandma, Grandad and Uncle Liam to do a memory walk for Shaun. About three hundred people turned up to walk from where Shaun lived as a child with his parents, Maggie and John, to his house more than a mile away down the hill.

It is heart-breaking how such a tragedy manages to bring together, many who have not seen one another in years. It would have been Shaun's thirty-ninth birthday.

The Government announced that we will fully return to Plan A on 27th January following the success of the booster vaccination programmes.

## 20th January 2022

It is now no longer official medical advice for teachers and pupils to wear face coverings in classrooms.

Stalling and messing around, instead of getting ready for nursery, is becoming an almost daily occurrence. We had to laugh, however, this morning when, instead of putting your uniform on, you laid it out on your bedroom floor. *Look! I've made a person!* you proudly declared.

At breakfast, you were that excited by the 'no sugar' syrup I had bought that you got a tape measure out to find out the height of the bottle. *It is ninety-nine quid!* you reported, inventing a new unit of measurement!

**25th January 2022**

Almost all of the house is packed up into boxes. The cases are ready to take on holiday in two weeks' time. You are probably wondering what it going on. Xander definitely does not have a clue what is going on!

You have previously said that you do not want to move house. The uncertainty of the situation is perhaps troubling you, which is ironic considering you have survived a pandemic. Whilst this house holds many fantastic memories for us as a family, our new home is where the majority of your childhood will now be enjoyed.

Before bed, you changed your mind and said you wanted to move house. *This house is rubbish.* Oh how fickle you can be!

There has been a change to the Covid-19 travel rules which means that people who have received both doses of the vaccine do not have to complete a Covid-19 test when returning from abroad.

**27th January 2022**

The last full day in our first family home.

I took the afternoon off work to help Mummy finish off packing and then I collected you from nursery. We took Quartz to Darcie and Ralphie's house as they are looking after him until we move into our new home.

Our last supper was a Chinese takeaway and I enjoyed my first alcoholic drink in 116 days.

Your last bedtime story was *The Snail and the Whale*, one that you have had so many times you now practically read to us!

## 28th January 2022

Moving day! Nana Roz arrived early to help. After breakfast, we walked round to Mrs Arain's house to give her family some flowers as a thank you for being great neighbours. The memories of those early months in lockdown, playing football in the garden, talking to them over the fence and being spoilt with chocolate and cars, are ones that we, as your parents, will cherish forever. You wondered what all the fuss was about as Mrs Arain, Mummy and I became emotional, hugging and saying goodbye.

As you left your old home for the last time, you said, *I'm never going to go into this house again.* Finality, delivered in nine words by a four-year-old!

The move ran relatively smoothly as we had already taken a lot of our belongings to our new home. Once the removal men had finished, Mummy and I waited outside the front of our empty former home and handed the keys to the new owners.

After exactly 480 weeks there, we were officially homeless. Everything is in place to move into our new home when we get back from holiday at the end of February.

# EPILOGUE

**25th February 2022**
Today we moved into our new house. Lots of work has been completed over the last few days to enable us to move in.

Uncle Liam, Auntie Emma, Darcie and Ralphie were our first visitors. They brought Quartz back, having looked after him for four weeks. Darcie approved of the place, opining, *I want to move to this house because it is beautiful!* You are quickly getting used to having to take your slippers off before you walk on the new carpets. We should have, perhaps, told you that the downstairs toilet was not yet functional before you weed in it!

Xander and Ralphie did very well to sleep through the noise of you and Darcie playing with dinosaurs in the playroom. You are really pleased with the dinosaur décor in your bedroom and it was only right that *Tyrannosaurus Drip* was your first bedtime story in your new home. Xander snored away in his cot in his bedroom across the landing, his first night sleeping alone.

\*

Almost two years ago, the country entered an unprecedented lockdown. Everyone, extremely naively in retrospect, thought that this would last for a few weeks. Writing this book was supposed to be a short project and here we are, 704 days later.

It is fitting that, as the book comes to a close, we are starting a new and exciting chapter as a family. The journey you have been on, your little brother Xander has not even begun. We hope that he never has to experience a pandemic.

The world is a place of fascinating wonder, but it can also be dangerous and cruel. Only yesterday, Russia declared war on Ukraine, an independent, sovereign European country.

The pandemic has been disruptive and difficult at times. As a family we have come out of it with little damage. No one close to us has been lost to the devastating virus that has caused so much hurt to millions of people worldwide. For that, we are thankful.

Without the pandemic, you would not have this loving, heart-warming and, some might say, humorous account of your life during the period. You were a toddler, a shade over two years old, in March 2020. Now you are very much a funny, cheeky, bright and affectionate little boy.

Our Little Man, it has been my pleasure!

# ABOUT THE AUTHOR

I am a public servant with more than fifteen years' experience working in the sector. With a background in Criminology, Social Work and Freelance Journalism, I have always harboured an ambition to be a published author. I do not claim to be an expert in Microbiology but I suppose I learned as much about viruses as the next person when writing this book.

When I was not writing *A Toddler's Tale: Life In Lockdown*, I spent my time playing golf, running and watching football in empty stadiums on television.

This is my debut book, centred around the life of my eldest child Noah throughout the Covid-19 pandemic.

I live in the North West of England with my wife Stacie and our three boys – Noah, Xander and Luca. Our rabbits, Marble and Quartz, did not live to see the book through to publication. Neither did the fish.

This book is printed on paper from sustainable sources managed under the Forest Stewardship Council (FSC) scheme.

It has been printed in the UK to reduce transportation miles and their impact upon the environment.

For every new title that Troubador publishes, we plant a tree to offset $CO_2$, partnering with the More Trees scheme.

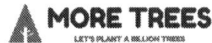

For more about how Troubador offsets its environmental impact, see www.troubador.co.uk/sustainability-and-community